Seven Ways To Make Running *Not Suck*

Mark Knoblauch PhD

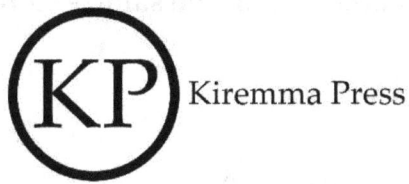

(KP) Kiremma Press

Printed in the United States of America

Disclaimer: This book is not intended as a substitute for the medical advice of licensed medical professionals. The reader should regularly consult his or her physician in any matter relating to his/her health and particularly with respect to any symptoms that may require diagnosis of a medical attention. Furthermore, The methods described within this book are the author's personal thoughts and opinions. As such, they are not intended to be a definitive set of instructions for you to follow precisely. You may discover there are other methods and materials to accomplish the same end result.

www.authorMK.com

ISBN: 978-1-7320674-0-0

This book is dedicated to anyone who makes the effort to run, whether it be for the health benefits or to ultimately win the race.

Table of Contents

Table of Contents

Introduction

If you are a runner, you'll likely agree that running can induce quite a split personality in many of us. On the one hand, we love the feeling that running can bring and we take pride in knowing that with every run we are improving our health. However, running can also induce feelings of dread or misery as we push through the physical exertion that running requires. Or we might have experienced all too often the guilt we feel after sleeping in rather than going for an early-morning run. Given the benefits that we all know running can bring, it is important that we maximize the opportunities we have that allow us to go running. To do this, we have to also recognize the threats that we can encounter which serve to dampen our desire to go for a run. For example, lack of motivation, weather, or injury can all play a role in suppressing any desire to run. Furthermore, fatigue or equipment issues such as poor running shoes can serve to make our runs miserable. And being miserable will have little effect on helping us stay motivated to run.

As a runner myself for well over ten years I've had the opportunity to have many conversations with fellow runners, both new and experienced. What I noticed were that many of those conversations kept bringing up repeated topics regarding factors that impact running. As I looked deeper into those discussions I found a unique difference between the new and experienced runner groups. Those new to running often centered around issues related to *problems* with particular facets of running such as equipment or motivation. Conversely, discussions with experienced runners tended to bring up those same topics, but the content of the conversation focused more on how they *overcame* those same issues, such as finding a proper shoe, or how they have been successful at battling the heat. Over time it became evident that new or less experienced runners seemed to point out the difficulties with their runs while more seasoned runners experienced those same issues yet found ways to prevent those issues from impacting their runs.

As I began to think through the various topics that most runners discuss, I realized that a properly-designed book could take those issues and format them in a way that could be beneficial to runners of all types. New, experienced, young, old, professional, amateur – all can benefit if the information is presented in the right way. Therefore, I wrote this book with all runners in mind and endeavored to highlight several common factors that can negatively influence runners. My plan for this book is to highlight those areas so as to make you the runner more aware, in turn helping to maximize the enjoyment and minimize the misery that can be found in running. Whereas the topics covered in this book stem largely from my own personal conversations with runners over the years, what you'll read here is by no means all-inclusive. In fact, I hope that you work to find many more tips and tricks on how to improve your own running outside of what is covered in this book.

In reading this book, I hope that you find the material useful. Any bit of information that can help you continue to run and stay healthy is beneficial, and my intent in writing this book is that you are able to use some of the information in this book to maintain an enthusiasm for running that lasts for many years. I think that by combining the content of this book along with other books that focus on proper training and/or nutrition, you will become a well-rounded runner that has few, if any limitations.

With that being said, let's get started on our journey together to help you become a more informed and more motivated runner.

Chapter 1: Set realistic goals

If you have been running for a while, you may have noticed every so often that you began to feel stagnant, or wondered if all the effort you put into running is really worth it. Or, if you are just starting to engage in a fitness-centered lifestyle, you may not be sure why you're doing it other than you were simply told to 'start exercising'. Either way, congratulate yourself for taking the steps necessary to be healthy. If you are in fact just starting out, the key is to ensure that you *continue* on this path to being healthy.

Like anything we do, running has days when it's fun and days when it's not so fun. The key is to maximize the 'fun' days in order to help push you through the not so fun days. One of the best ways to do this is to establish a goal and then spend your efforts working towards that goal. When you see progress toward your goal – or even better yet, accomplishment of that goal – the motivation you have to press on can be inspiring. To help you both get and stay inspired, this chapter focuses on how goal setting can help you in your quest to enjoy running, as well as examine a few different goal options that may help your runs become more productive.

What is a goal

A goal could be defined as a target of one's ambition, or a desired result. We all have goals in some way or another whether they are work-related, family-related, grand in scale like achieving an early retirement, or small in scope such as when we strive to make it to work on time. Goals provide motivation, and in strenuous activity events such as running, motivation can be a necessary tool to ensure that you stay on track. Fitness-related goals are especially beneficial, because at worst, whether you actually achieve them or not you are contributing towards improving your health. And as your health improves you will likely find that many of your goals – even perhaps some not specifically related to health – begin to change over time, such as trying to reach a higher fitness level, longer race, or faster finish.

Benefits of Goal setting

When you set goals, you establish a new challenge for yourself. For some of us, a challenge provides much-needed motivation to keep working towards a specific outcome. As an example, imagine if your physician recommends you to lose weight. Assuming you've had a lifestyle rife with inactivity, there's little chance that you will be enthused to engage in an exercise program to lose weight in order to become healthier. It's just not in your mindset and you have little motivation to do so given that it was simply a recommendation from your physician. However, if your insurance company will reduce your insurance rates by 15% if you get your cholesterol levels below a certain value, you now have a financial incentive, and a type of indirect challenge, to lose the weight.

In both situations, you don't *have* to lose weight or lower your cholesterol, but you may be motivated enough to try to do so. While such a request from your physician or your insurance company may be the challenge you need, running is no different when it comes to setting goals. Some may find the desire to complete a 5K, or a half-marathon, or a marathon to be their challenge. Either way, once committing to a race there is usually an inherent motivation to accomplish the goal. You might even be a runner already, competing at one level but knowing deep down that you have the capability of achieving greater success. When it comes to goal setting, it doesn't matter if your ultimate goal is to engage in a new, active lifestyle or simply improve upon your abilities – almost everyone can benefit from establishing a goal.

Keeping you on track

One of the best things about goal setting is that it provides you a pathway for at least the near – if not long-term – future. With a goal in mind, you have an endpoint and can then begin to work backwards to develop a realistic schedule that will help you achieve that goal. For example, if you have a goal to run a 5K, you know that your current status as a couch potato will allow that goal to happen. You need to do the things that will allow your body to run 3.1 miles without fatiguing to the point that it cannot continue on, all within the available time that remains prior to the 5K. Whereas your fitness level is not anywhere close to that goal as a couch potato, it lets you know that for a certain amount of time – the time you have remaining before your 5K – you must continually improve in order to reach that goal. Therefore, if the

5K is two weeks away and you cannot run 100 meters without stopping, your goal was probably a bit unrealistic as your timeline ultimately will not allow the goal to be achieved.

Keeping you motivated

It's easy to procrastinate when you're doing something 'just to do it'. If your plan is to go for a three or five mile run every day, a particularly busy work day may make you more inclined to skip the run if there is no goal. After all, if you're not necessarily working to improve your run time or lose weight, skipping a run has no real consequence and results in nothing more than the fact that you failed to burn extra calories on that particular day. Procrastination can be rampant in the exercise world. After all, without a firm goal it's not always motivating to perform sweaty work for 30 to 60 minutes or more when you could instead enjoy a nap.

We all would love to take the path of least resistance, but unfortunately when it comes to exercise, taking the easy way out can have consequences. Short-term consequences of simply skipping a run may end up as nothing more than feeling guilty or perhaps not sleeping particularly well that night. Long-term consequences, however –

brought about by repetitively skipping runs – may induce weight gain, cause fatigue, or induce other health-related fatigue. As those factors worsen in response to continuing to skip workouts, we may become less and less motivated to continue running at all.

Setting a goal helps keep you on-target and gives you a reason why it is important not to procrastinate. If you have a race goal in the future, or a weight-loss goal, the consequences associated with skipping a run can be much more evident. I myself have fallen victim to having a lack of motivation. After completing a marathon or triathlon that I had been training months for, there was little motivation in the days and weeks afterwards to continue running. Because the big event that required months of training and healthy eating had now passed, I fell into the mindset that I could finally eat what I wanted, skip a workout if so desired, and generally laze around. Later, however, I clearly suffered the consequences of those decisions once starting back up on my next training goal, for it took me weeks to recover from the down time I accumulated during my minimal training period. Without an ensuing goal lined up, I clearly lacked the motivation to train. This in turn cost me additional time to get back to an acceptable level when training for a subsequent race.

To avoid any subsequent detriments in my training schedule, I began to schedule future events (e.g. marathon, triathlon, etc.) before any currently scheduled event had occurred.

Because you will likely be more focused if you have a goal, there will be less time for activities which do not lead you directly towards your established goal. For example, if you sign up for a 10K, when faced with the option of watching television or going for a run, you will likely be more motivated to run as doing so will contribute to the preparation for your race. Similarly, if you have a training goal in mind you may have a more directed and focused run, in which you gain a particular benefit such as an improved pace. Otherwise, you may just feel that you need to go out and "get a run in" with no real direction or purpose. By setting a goal, you are likely going to be more focused on achieving that goal, in turn becoming more willing to put in the effort to reach that goal.

Barriers to achieving goals

Setting a goal is not the difficult part of any plan; rather, achieving that goal is the hard part. One of the key factors of something being a goal is that it will take a significant amount of effort on your part to accomplish, and that effort will result in something that you can likely consider an accomplishment. Unfortunately, as we are all well-aware, not every goal is reached.

As a runner you must accept that barriers exist which can prevent you from reaching your goals. Some barriers are external, or beyond your reach – injury, a new job assignment, or an unexpected illness. In most cases, these barriers will pass and you can resume pursuit of your goal. Other times, barriers can come from within. These internal barriers can be the hardest to overcome because we set the barrier ourselves. For example, lack of motivation can be an internal barrier. If you are not motivated, such as in a case where you are running just to make someone else (e.g. spouse) happy, you are not likely motivated and will therefore have less of a likelihood that you will accomplish your goal(s). Similarly, sleep can serve to become a barrier. If you sleep in once from a morning run, you will be more likely to sleep in again as you found that you could get away with it without much consequence. Therefore, surely not much harm will come from sleeping in twice, right? And so the process starts.

Remember, barriers are just that – events that get in the way of your goals. Exercise as well as running itself have plenty of barriers. Next we will discuss some of the more common and general internal barriers. This list is by no means exhaustive. Rather, it helps, outline the most common internal barriers to success and can hopefully serve to help you recognize internal barriers so that you can better prevent their occurrence.

Excessively difficult goals

Be careful in setting goals that are too high, as failing to reach them could have drastic consequences such as effectively shutting down your desire to continue running. Using a previous example, if you are a couch potato and set a goal of running a marathon, what is your timeframe? Some may say that a year or more is necessary to reach a goal like that. But if after two months you are struggling to run a 5K, a marathon looks much more daunting – so much that you may be inclined to quit. Therefore, make sure that any goal you set is in fact *realistic*. For example, running a marathon is fine to set as a goal – it's just probably not the initial goal you should set if you have not been running for very long. Instead, develop a set of mini-goals that will help you reach your overall goal. For example, our couch potato could set a progressive set of races as separate goals – completing a 5K, 10K, and half marathon initially.

Perhaps then he or she will be able to focus on completing a marathon. As we have discussed, goals are motivating, so even achieving the small goals will help motivate you on to accomplishing the major goal.

Comparing your results to that of others

If you are running with a group or at least a partner, you have already taken a step towards ensuring that you are on a path to achieving your goal. Engaging with a running partner or social group can be outstanding for helping you achieve a running goal. However, running with others can also inhibit your own goals if you compare your personal results to those of someone else. It's easy to *want* to compare your own results to those of another runner, given that in a running group everyone is effectively participating in the same activity. But there are so many factors at play between what you are trying to do versus what everyone else is trying to accomplish. As a result, you cannot realistically make a direct comparison between your own results and those of another. For example, you would have to equate age, fitness level, metabolism, run history, body fat percentage, equipment types, and probably body weight before even beginning to expect have the same results as another person in your group. If that person you are comparing yourself against is five years younger than you, you should automatically disqualify yourself from expecting similar performance gains (e.g. pace, distance, etc.) given the known effect that age can have on those performance-related measures. If you are the same age but have 8% higher body fat percentage, or have been running for 1/3 of the years as the other person, you cannot allow yourself to expect the same results. Only when relevant running-related factors have been accounted for (and are equal) can you being to draw comparisons between yourself and another runner. But, establishing those factors still might not capture enough information to allow you to judge your results against those of another.

Impatience

Biology does not work at society's pace. If you want to lose 10 pounds of fat before your friend's wedding in two weeks, you should expect to fail. Similarly, if you want to be able to run a half-marathon a month after starting a training program, again – expect to fail. We have to give our body time to adapt to the demands that we expect of it. If we don't, the physical changes necessary to reach our goal cannot happen. If you had a goal of waking up by 6a.m. ten days in a row, doing so does not require a physiological change to the body. Rather, it requires only a bit of discipline and remembering to set an alarm clock. Expecting physiological changes in the body in the same time frame, though, is not realistic.

Fitness goals aren't just about setting the goal – we have to also allow our body to make the adaptations necessary to achieve that goal. For example, we can easily say that we want to lose 10 pounds. Most likely we are referring to the fact that we want to lose 10 pounds of *fat* in two weeks. Unfortunately, we simply cannot realistically lose 10 pounds of fat in two weeks (you could theoretically lose 10 pounds of *weight* in terms of 'water weight', but it will come back quickly) because the process by which our body breaks down fat and utilizes it for energy does not happen that fast. Therefore, like we discussed earlier in this chapter, goals we set have to be realistic. Impatience will have no effect, as our bodies are bound by what biology dictates. When it comes to weight loss or improvements in our run performance that are the result of physiological changes within our body, we just can't 'speed up' the process; rather, we can only give it the best opportunity to occur by reducing our caloric intake or participating in a proper training plan. A more realistic time frame for losing weight would be – at minimum – six to eight weeks. Even then, a high level of discipline combined with exercise would be required.

Pushing yourself too hard

Motivation can be a great thing, but if you're not careful it can have the potential to lead to your downfall. If you try too hard to meet your goal(s) by running more than you should, you can experience one of the two most successful goal-killers in the running world – burnout or injury. Burnout happens when you lose motivation and realize that even your personal goal no longer seems worthwhile. Burnout can be quite hard to overcome, as it is internal in nature, and without clear and continued motivation you have no desire or need to progress further. Often, burnout comes from pushing yourself too hard. For example, adopting a mindset that 'one run per day is good, so two is better' may mentally fatigue you to the point that you have no desire to run anymore. To avoid burnout, you have to be aware of the chance that burnout can occur and work to pull yourself back from continuing on a path that increases its likelihood of occurrence. Being excited to go for a run is great and is a very encouraging behavior to have, but suppressing the desire to get in multiple runs per day and instead limiting yourself to one good run a day can help reduce the risk of burnout.

A second consequence of pushing yourself too hard is injury. When it comes to our body's physiology, it's quite simple to understand – if you overwork the body, you increase the risk of injury significantly. The body is designed to be stressed, but every part of your body has a limit, and with running-related activity it is usually the bones, muscles, or joints that give in first. Because these tissues need to recover from *every* run you do, if you push them too hard – such as might occur with intense or excessively long runs – the tissues will likely break down. The breakdown may not be rapid and may even be undetectable until it becomes severe. If this occurs, you may not realize you are injured until you discover that the strange pain you feel in your shin is actually a rather severe stress fracture.

When it comes to scheduling your workouts, remember this – the body gets stronger by being subjected to a controlled level of mechanical stress such as occurs with proper amounts of running. To get stronger, the body has to be able to repair the microscopic damage that occurs during every workout. With this repair comes overall stronger tissue that we see as a trained body. If instead another mechanical stress comes along (such as another excessively long run) before the repairs are complete, that additional stress will cause further damage. Over time, this process triggers a breakdown of the tissue which can result in chronic injury that will prevent you from pursuing and accomplishing your running goals.

Listening to the naysayers

There are naysayers to some degree in pretty much everyone's life. This may be a voice deep inside your own head or it may be a friend or family member. To reach your goals you have to be able to block out the negative and focus on the positive. You will likely know someone who constantly questions why you run. Quite frankly, it doesn't matter why you run. A better question might be: why don't *they* run? The fact is, you run because you want to, and at the least you are improving your health. As such, it's quite difficult to justify any reason as to why you should not run.

If you encounter naysayers – including those that exist in your own mind – you have to realize that the positives outweigh the negatives when it comes to running-related goals. Your particular goal may be to simply run three times a week, or finish a race;

ultimately, it doesn't matter what your goal is. If you do not have a close circle of support for your running goals, you need to find an outlet that will allow you the resources you need to pursue and achieve your goal. This may require joining a running group or an online social media site, or in some cases it may require simply being left alone to run.

In conclusion

Whatever it takes, recognize that running has a wealth of benefits. As such, staying engaged in running can help you live a healthier life. Goal setting can play a significant role in helping to keep you on track in your running activity, and can serve as a type of motivation for you to continue to pursue running as a way to enhance your health and fitness. However, it is also important to ensure that the goals you set for yourself are realistic and can occur within a reasonable time frame, for if your goals were not designed properly they can end up destroying your motivation and potentially ending your desire to run. In the next chapter we'll look at some of the other various motivators along with goal-setting that you can use to help keep you engaged in your running.

Chapter 2: Find your motivators

Running is a viable way to get out of the house and into the great outdoors. Even more important is that running is an outstanding mechanism for improving your health. And when your health improves, the motivation to continue engaging in the responsible activity will almost certainly increase as well. Ask anyone who is on a diet if losing a pound or two on the scale is exciting, and you'll certainly get a resounding 'yes!'. As we discussed in the previous chapter, the success of accomplishing even the initial phases of your goal, such as one pound of weight loss out of an overall anticipated goal of 20 pounds, can be extremely motivating and give you the energy you need to continue on in pursuit of your goal.

Running is no different when it comes to having a need to stay motivated. Hopefully, all runners have a goal of some kind that they are working towards. These goals do not necessarily have to be to get faster, or to run farther. Running-related goals can be as simple as 'run five times in one week'. It is the accomplishment of a goal – and many times, the motivation to achieve the goal – that can supply the incentive and enthusiasm to pursue the next goal.

For anyone who has been running for an extended amount of time, they will almost certainly recall a time when it was a little harder to find the energy and drive to get a run started. For some it may have been getting out of bed early in the morning, or perhaps the temperature had dipped enough to convince them that staying in a warm house would make more sense. These kinds of excuses will come up, but they are relatively short-term in duration. If you are anything like me, the day-long guilt that occurs after turning off my alarm and going back to sleep (instead of getting in my early-morning workout) is depressing enough to ensure that I don't allow it to happen again the next day. Nevertheless, short-term effects (e.g. guilt) that can occur after skipping a workout are not particularly problematic. In fact, everyone should take a day off every few days or so to allow the body ample time to recover. The bigger problem is *long-term* lack of motivation, which can ultimately terminate a running program and send the runner right back to the couch. Therefore, anything that you can do to stay motivated to run should be utilized to its full effect.

Music

Going on a short or long run can be fun, but without an adequate distraction some runners are left with nothing but the thoughts in their head. For runners like myself, heading out with just my thoughts can be productive. I switched gradually from using an MP3 player on my runs to eventually going without any sort of music. While difficult at first, I eventually found time to 'think' on my runs. In fact, the idea for this book was conceived on a run, and by the end of that same run I had several of the chapter ideas worked out. However, going without music may not be for everyone and, depending on the day, I may elect to put in the earbuds and listen to my playlist on a run. You may find that music (or another distractor such as an e-book) during your helps to take your mind off of the physical exertion of the run. If a constant focus on the required exertion could be viewed as a detriment to you accomplishing your run, then music should definitely be a part of your running activity.

If you do in fact utilize music on your runs, what happens if the music is unavailable, such as due to having a dead battery – does the run get cancelled? If so, you have become too dependent upon your music device as you lose all motivation to run if the music is not available. Try to work in a few runs, even short ones, in which you do nothing but listen to the sounds around you. There is a sort of inherent beauty to be had in listening to the sound of nature on a run which can serve as its own distraction if you allows it. That in itself is my purpose for running without music in the mornings, as I take solace in the sounds around me at that time of day. Furthermore, you should be aware that some races do not allow the use of portable listening devices as they can distract the runner from potential hazards such as a passing runner. If you have become dependent upon your music device but then find out at your race that you cannot use it, such news may negatively affect your motivation to continue the race. Therefore, be sure that you can in fact run without the requirement of having a portable music device with you.

Music devices now come in several shapes and sizes. Gone are the days of the bulky cassette player that provided no real convenience on a run. Some runners prefer to have their cell phone play music while strapped to their arm, which is particularly useful in the event that they need to make an emergency call for something such as an injury. Personally, I have found success with my small MP3 player that I can clip onto my waistband. By threading the headphone wires inside my shirt I can avoid the annoyance that comes with the wires flopping around. Regardless of how you design your personal setup, if music is your motivation – use it when you can.

Social support

If you are a 'loner' like me and prefer to run on your own, great for you. In doing so you can avoid having to schedule your runs according to the availability of a partner, or rearrange your run schedule in the event that your partner cannot make it to the run or has to reschedule at the last minute. Not all runners are loners, though, and some prefer the support of other runners to keep them going. If this is you, look for ways to engage socially with other runners in your area. For example, joining a local running group is probably the best way to find other runners in your area, and given the amount of runners often present at these groups, you are likely to find someone with a similar ability or running schedule as you. Many runners feel that joining a running group can help them stay accountable by making it more difficult to skip a scheduled run, almost feeling as if the group run is dependent upon them. Getting to the group run is often the difficult part, as once you arrive and experience the camaraderie of the group, the run itself becomes an afterthought.

Social media has done wonders for connecting runners of all kinds. Whether it be a social media group or a phone app, the instant access that you have via social media is a great way to get a run in with a partner or group. I have both joined and started my own social media fitness group, and the speed at which others in my area joined was amazing. Within hours people were posting times that they planned to run in the area, at the same time inviting anyone else to join in if interested. Expect that once you have a few passionate members in your group you will soon be attending shopping trips and weekend cookouts together, with the topic of running working its way into the event's conversations at some point. Social support is not only motivating but it can also help to build lifelong friendships.

Internet

There's no doubt that we live in the information age. We have a wealth of learning materials and tools at our disposal thanks to the internet, and as a runner you should be taking full advantage of it all. Simply typing "running tips" or some similar phrase into an internet search can bring you a wealth of relevant information that will certainly be of benefit to your running. There is so much information, in fact, that you can tailor your search results to the information most specific to your own needs, such as that focused on your training level, area of the country, gender, age, fitness level, or even preferred type of running equipment.

If you want to know if the running-related information is valuable, I can tell you without question that it is. You will have to be able to weed out some of the bad information, such as that which is more focused on selling you a particular product, but there is a mind-blowing amount of helpful information out there to improve your running. Given the simple, no-cost nature of that information, you must ensure that you take advantage of it all.

If, for example, you are a new runner, I would suggest finding a website and/or message board geared toward helping new runners be successful. Or, if you have some experience under your belt, you might find tips for matching your running style to the type of running equipment that you need. Regardless of your interest, if you look hard enough on the internet you will find the answer.

In some cases you can find information straight from those who know best – the professionals. Many blogs, tips, and/or web pages are posted by highly successful runners that want to help those getting started in the sport. Some even allow you personalized information or tips, though often at a particular price. Regardless of how you get the information, spend the required time on the internet searching for information that is relevant to you, as you will undoubtedly find what you are looking for.

In conclusion

Given the individual differences that we all have, it is certain that we will also have differences in what motivates us. Regardless of what your particular motivator is, if it helps to get you up and running, use it. At the same time, don't allow that particular motivator to be the *only* reason that you run. If that happens, you will likely avoid running if your motivator (e.g. a partner, music, etc.) is not available. Therefore spend the effort to get in a few runs that do not require your motivator so as to ensure that you are still able to run. But during the other times, take advantage of your motivator as it will likely make for a more enjoyable time while on your runs.

Chapter 3: Establish your baselines

No matter if you have been running for years on your own or are just now ready to start, you have to know where you have been in terms of ability in order to determine if you are making progress. Even those runners who like to run as a means to get out of the house are certain to appreciate the benefits that running can have on one's health. Regardless of whether you are trying to positively impact your health or you want to improve performance factors such as pace or distance, in order to determine if you are making positive progress you need to monitor your progress over time with measurable data. Yes, even something as simple as running can be infiltrated by statistics. And as a runner, you need to develop the mindset that statistics are going to be your best tool for determining the effectiveness of your running program. In this chapter, we'll look at a few different baseline measures including those affecting weight, running, and blood markers. As you repeat these measures over time, you will be able to see whether the values change favorably or non-favorably, in turn allowing you to determine the effectiveness of your running program.

Determine your variable of interest

You might think that running is all about pace and distance. In a way, that is correct, and both of those are measurable aspects of running. However, it is likely that you will also want to know if you are impacting certain other health-related aspects involved with running. Such aspects can include change in body weight or percent body fat, or certain blood markers such as cholesterol. For example, have you wondered if your running is lowering your blood pressure, or if you are losing muscle or fat? Similarly, have you increased your pace after one month of running? These are all measurable variables related to running, and it is important that you establish the current level of the variable you are interested in (e.g. body weight, cholesterol level, etc.) so that you can measure change over time.

Another factor to consider is whether a particular outcome is *intended*. For example, longtime or competitive runners may run 10 miles a day and not lose a single pound of fat over six months. Most likely, with their level of body fat and overall fitness level they probably do not *want* to lose fat. As such, their runs will be focused on improving race-related factors such as pace and will likely not be intended to result in weight loss. Conversely, a new runner may be able to run two miles a day, and with a careful diet might lose six pounds in a month.

A change in a particular variable of interest is impacted by several factors such as total running time, intensity, and perhaps even diet. Oftentimes, you can impact a single variable of interest by adjusting one particular aspect of running. For example, if you are interested in targeting body fat you will typically have better results by completing longer, slower-runs as compared to short runs at a high pace. However, if it is your intent to improve your run pace, it will necessitate a faster running speed that may not allow you to burn as much body fat as you would at a slower pace.

The importance of baselines

For many of us, seeing results is a tremendous motivator. However, without a reliable comparison, the results can mean nothing. Imagine that you have been running for six months and after those six months you 'feel' great. Of course feeling great is a positive outcome of your efforts spent running. But, what might be the actual reason that you feel great? If after six months of running I were to show you a chart that reveals seven pounds of weight loss, you would likely be inclined to keep running. However, if I showed you a chart revealing that you *gained* seven pounds during that time despite 'feeling' great, would all of the effort spent running be worth it? Possibly not. In fact, you may start to wonder why you're running at all since you know running is supposed to result in weight loss despite the fact that your weight is in fact increasing. Had you been monitoring your weight *during* those six months rather than only at the end, you may have noticed a trend such as weight loss or gain over time. Revealing a trend would in turn allow you to determine if your program was effective, and would allow you to make adjustments as necessary or perhaps revamp the program if you are not getting the results you want. But if you do not record a baseline, you have no indication of where your current variable of interest is at compared to where it was at the start. And without any data to follow over time, you have no idea as to whether you are making progress as a result of your running activity.

Data is simple to keep track of. Just find a valid tool that *accurately* measures the factor you are interested in, and then record the results over time.

For example, if you look at a clock as you leave the house and then again when you return, that's not the best method for determining your run time. You may have stretched in the driveway, or waited at a couple of red lights which were not accounted for when measured by "total time out of the house". However, if you use a digital stopwatch, you could start the timer when you exit your driveway and stop it when you return. Furthermore, each time you cease running activity – such as at a stoplight – you can stop the timer. This allows for much more accurate timing, which will allow you to look at trends over time, even when your runs might differ by only seconds per week.

Much like the earlier example regarding weight loss, if you have been running consistently for six months and you find out that your total cholesterol level increased by 40 points, are you going to be happy about that? Probably not, especially given the fact that you are likely running for the sole reason of becoming healthier. But with the elevated cholesterol, are you in fact becoming healthier? You may feel like you can run farther or feel as though you have more energy, but "feeling" anything isn't really a measurable outcome. Cholesterol level is measurable, and if your test results show an increase in total cholesterol after months of running, something probably is not right. It may be that you simply need to alter your diet in addition to your running, but without knowing what your baseline values are when you first start a running program, you'll have no comparison.

What if, for example, after four months of running you go in for your initial cholesterol check and find that the value is 270mg/dl. You might be encouraged, assuming that the value after four months of running is certainly lower that what it was when you started running. But, without a baseline to compare the current value to, you have no comparison and therefore should not assume that the current value represents a decrease in your cholesterol since you started running. Who knows, it may be 30mg/dl higher than when you started running. The only real comparison you would be able to make is to take another cholesterol test a few months later and then compare that test's results to your four-month test. If that test shows a decrease in cholesterol from 270mg/dl, it is evidence suggesting that your running program is working. But, if the value is higher than 270mg/dl, you would have to decide if your cholesterol has always been going up since you started running, or if it has just gone up since the four-month test, which you will not know without having the initial test values from when you started running. Again, establishing a baseline allows you to see trends over time as the test is repeated, and if your values go up regardless of your running activity, you'll know that you need to either alter your exercise program or perhaps re-evaluate your diet.

Get your physical

Even in the event you are already actively running, if you haven't had a thorough physical examination from your physician, get one. And if you are already getting your annual checkups but plan to start running, let your physician know so that he or she can determine whether you're ready for physical exertion-type activity. An annual physical can be one of the best things you can do for yourself at any age, not just when you are over 40 years old.

As a runner, your physical exam will not only allow your physician to determine if your body is physically ready to exercise, it will also help establish several baseline values that you can track over time. Depending on your physician, your physical might record your weight, blood pressure, and if you or your physician request it, perhaps even a "blood panel" which will let you know the values of several important blood factors such as cholesterol, glucose, and sodium. These factors are important not only for determining your overall health, but they are also important to monitor as you exercise over time. Running can influence each of these values, and having a valid, reliable baseline measure will provide the foundation to establish whether your running program is effective for a particular variable.

Understanding body composition baselines

If you're relatively new to running, there's a good chance that you are running to either lose weight or perhaps maintain a particular body weight. If so, you are likely wanting to know how much fat is on your body, which is a measurable variable. Or, you may be running with the intent of losing weight, which is also a measurable variable, though somewhat less specific in what the "weight" is comprised of. Therefore, the key is to determine the makeup of any 'weight' that is lost – specifically, if the lost weight is fat, muscle, or perhaps even fluid lost through sweating.

Weight

Unfortunately, the determinant of body weight – the dreaded 'scale' – gets a bad rap. It shouldn't invoke the mild terror that it often does, but people still fear the scale regardless. It has such an unfortunate job, sitting there calmly and every once in a while reporting accurate values, yet ultimately it is despised for simply telling the truth. Quite simply, a scale just measures how much force the earth is pulling you down with, which generates what we know as *weight*. Somehow it seems as though that force is always more than we want it to be. But why do we get so upset about our weight? It's just a number, right? Well, it's 'supposed' to be just a number. If anything, the scale's reported weight value can be *good*, in that it tells us whether what we're doing is or isn't working yet we despise it nonetheless.

Although the scale is simply reporting a number – our weight – there are in fact certain conditions that can influence our weight that have nothing to do with weight loss. As such, it is important to control for those conditions so that we can be sure that any change between a particular value and our baseline value is in fact due to true weight loss. Therefore, we'll look at these conditions specifically.

To measure any change in your weight, which we certainly hope is a positive change, you want to make sure that you are consistent from one weigh-in to the next. If not, you will see wild fluctuation in your weight, which could induce great joy if you see weight loss or significant frustration with evidence of weight gain. To control for this, be sure that you weigh yourself under the same conditions from one day to the next.

1) Always wear the same amount and type of clothing when you weigh yourself. Obtaining your weight in heavy clothing such as jeans and a sweatshirt one day and then in workout attire a couple of days later will automatically affect your results by a pound or more. Heavier clothes for the follow-up weigh-in will always add weight, while wearing light clothes will result in a lower weight, even if your true weight did not change at all. Consequently, appearing to weigh less at a second weigh-in due to wearing lighter clothes will certainly be followed with a subsequent 'heavier' weigh-in if the third scale reading is taken when wearing substantially more clothing.

2) Always weigh yourself after consuming identical amounts of food and water as was consumed previously. This could also mean consuming *no* food or drink if that is what occurred during a previous weigh-in. For example, if you get up one morning and weigh yourself immediately, but three days later weigh yourself after drinking two

eight-ounce cups of coffee, you have automatically added one pound of weight to the scale's readout. Automatically! And, if you have lost a pound of true weight during that same time, the pound added back from the coffee will make it appear as though you have had no effect on weight resulting from your exercise.

Another important point when it comes to food and scales is to think of food as weight. A healthy soup or a salad are both excellent meals when on a weight-loss diet, but a soup will likely add more weight *to the scale's readout* than the salad. Therefore, think of the foods you are eating when you weigh yourself, and for a truly accurate scale reading, factor in the weight of the food when weighing. For example, weigh that bowl of spaghetti that you eat. Then, when you get on the scale be sure to *subtract* that amount of weight from the scale's readout.

3) Similar to the food you consume, be consistent when using the scale before or after using the restroom. If you wake up in the morning and immediately urinate before stepping on the scale, and then three days later weigh yourself before urinating, you could easily add a half-pound to a pound (or more) of weight to the second scale reading.

4) Don't forget to factor in exercise! When you work out strenuously, you sweat. Sweat has mass, so

it has weight. If you sweat a lot and don't replenish any sweat, you could easily weigh 2-3 pounds less after a workout than before. If you like to weigh yourself after workouts and don't first replenish the fluid lost through sweat, you can easily create false hope that you lost several pounds just from a long run. In reality, you may have burned through 1/3 pound of fat after a long run, but the scale makes it look as though you lost two, three, or more pounds.

If your workouts are consistent, meaning that you do the same workout every time, it is somewhat acceptable to weigh yourself after a workout because the amount of fluid lost should be relatively consistent. Thought the weight is not exactly correct on the scale, it will *always* have the same level of inconsistency, allowing you to observe the change over time. Understand, however, that changes in temperature or relative humidity (affecting sweat lost) or type of clothing worn (certain clothing fibers can absorb more fluid) can influence the value on a scale after a workout. Therefore, it is preferable that you weigh yourself *prior* to any workout so as to get both a consistent weight and your true weight.

5) Perhaps the most important of all these factors is to always – always – weigh yourself on the same scale. Some like myself will argue that it is more important to have a reliable weight reported rather

than a valid (i.e. accurate) value. If I get on a scale that is randomly off by anywhere from one to 15 pounds, I cannot trust any of the values that it reports. My weight on that scale may be 210 pounds, it may be reported as 225 pounds, or it may be 195 pounds, or anywhere in between. But, if a scale is *consistently* off by three pounds on the light side, I can rest assured that my weight on that particular scale is always going to be 207 pounds even though a truly calibrated scale says I'm 210 pounds. Therefore, you have to ensure that the scale you are using is reliable, which means that it gets a value consistently over time, even if that value is not actually correct. In a perfect world, the scale you use will be reliable *and* valid, and it is always nice to be able to weigh yourself on a scale that shows evidence of calibration. But depending on the setting you are in, having a truly accurate scale may not always be feasible.

One problem I have personally observed on several occasions is when someone records their weight at home, then goes to work or school and checks their weight again. This is about as *in*accurate of a way to measure weight over time as you can get. Even if there was truly no change in your weight, you are left up to the accuracy of each individual scale, which really ends up telling you nothing because you don't know which scale is correct. If you weigh yourself at home and get a value of 143, then drive to work and weigh 147 on the work scale, which value is correct? I would be willing to bet that you are suddenly more confident in the home scale given that it showed a lower weight. But, what if the home scale was three pounds off and the work scale was correct? As this example reveals, it is important to avoid the potential for an inaccurately measured change in your weight by always using the same scale.

Failure to be aware of the conditions listed above can negatively influence the value reported by your scale. If you go for a five-mile run and then weigh yourself afterwards, you'll certainly weigh less than before the run simply due to the loss of sweat. And, you might be wearing lighter clothing for your run. The next day – after consuming adequate fluid since your run that served to replenish the sweat lost during the run – the weight from those five miles' worth of sweat will be back on the scale's readout. You have thereby set up an opportunity for a bit of depression when you step on the scale only to see a much higher weight than was recorded the previous day after your run. Only when you stay true to the conditions listed above can any scale's reported change in weight be considered to be true weight gain or loss. Failure to adhere to the principles that we just discussed about consistency between weigh-ins are in fact reason to throw out the value reported by the scale.

Percent body fat

The second important value to monitor when interested in losing weight is that of percent body fat. As we showed above, 'losing weight' involves simply stepping on a scale and seeing that the value is lower than a previous weigh-in. However, that value tells nothing about *where* the lost weight is coming from, and as we indicated, the weight could be simply due to water weight, clothing, or consumed food. Body composition, of which percent body fat is a factor, is a much more accurate way of determining where weight loss occurs in your body. A body composition measure tells you what percent of your body is composed of fat and what percent is "everything else" (e.g. muscle). Follow-up measures can then establish whether there has been any change in the amount of fat on your body after you have been engaged in your running program.

Your first thought may be that you don't want to know how much fat you have on you, but trust me, you do. Remember, if the scale reports that you have lost weight, you will want to know if that lost weight is from muscle mass or fat. Without having obtained a baseline measure of your body fat you won't know. If you're like most people you likely want to be losing body fat and not muscle. However, if a body composition analysis shows that a reduction in your weight is due to a loss of muscle mass rather than fat, you can counter that loss of muscle mass with a simple strength training program. Without knowing your body composition, you won't know where the loss is occurring.

There are several ways to measure body fat, and the specifics of each are beyond the scope of this book. The important thing to remember is to get a baseline measure as soon as you can, which will then allow you to measure subsequent changes in that value over time. Also understand that accuracy of the reported value generally diminishes as the cost of the equipment used to measure body composition decreases. One of the best body composition tools is the dual x-ray absorptiometry (DEXA) scan which simply requires you to lie down on a table and allow a scanner to pass over you. However, simple skinfold calipers can tell you viable information as well, as long as the person performing the test is trained on the technique. Other options include hydrostatic (underwater) weighing as well as the simple but not as reliable bioimpedance machines, which exist in many different styles (including home bathroom scales) and price ranges.

Aerobic Capacity

Your body's aerobic capacity is best measured through assessment of what is known as your VO2max. By definition, VO2max is known as *milliliters of oxygen per kilogram of body mass per minute,* but it can be described much simpler as the highest rate by which your cardiovascular system can transport oxygenated blood to the muscles effectively. If your body cannot transport adequate oxygen during exercise, fatigue sets in.

Over time, a good running program can be expected to increase your VO2max significantly. Endurance running has the most drastic effects, much more than can be gained with shorter, faster runs that are well-known for building speed. Increases in aerobic capacity occur through several modifications such as increasing how much blood is sent to your muscles, increasing the amount of blood vessels in your muscles, and increasing the amount of blood your heart pumps out with each beat, among other modifications.

Getting a baseline aerobic capacity measurement is not going to have much value if your goal is weight loss, but it will provide important information if you are looking to improve factors related to your running activity. If you have a high aerobic capacity despite doing no real physical activity, you likely have a tremendous capability for improvement in running factors such as pace or distance. Or, if your VO2max value is relatively low but you have significant body fat, you still have a lot of room for improvement in aerobic capacity (and therefore your ability to improve certain running factors) with an effective training plan and a well-designed diet.

Blood lactate

There are a wealth of running-related variables that you can measure to establish your baseline levels. While aerobic capacity is measured by analyzing the content of the air that you exhale during exercise, it is also possible to measure variables within the blood. One of the easiest markers (i.e. variables) is the blood lactate test. This is a simple test that requires only a small droplet of blood while you exercise on a treadmill. Lactate is a by-product of energy production in your body, and your muscle cells quickly neutralize the lactate and prevent it from affecting the acidity of the muscle tissue (which can trigger fatigue). If lactate is produced at a level that exceeds the muscle's ability to neutralize the lactate, the muscle will start sending the excess lactate to the blood. We can then observe (through analysis of a blood droplet) changes in blood lactate levels and determine what pace is too fast for your muscles to adequately neutralize generated lactate (known as the 'lactate threshold') and thereby know what running pace you should maintain to delay fatigue.

If you want to know the most effective pace to run at for your particular fitness level, a baseline blood lactate test is recommended. As your fitness improves, your muscles develop an improved capacity to neutralize lactate, thereby allowing you to exercise at a higher rate before lactate becomes a factor. By measuring the change in your running pace at which blood lactate concentrations begin to accumulate, you will be able to see over time if your running activity is setting you up to improve your running pace.

The lactate threshold test has been around for many years and is quite simple to complete. You will begin slowly on a piece of exercise equipment such as a treadmill or bike, after which the speed will be increased at specific intervals. In conjunction with these intervals, you will have a small droplet of blood taken from a fingertip which will then be collected and analyzed for lactate. This value will be plotted on a graph. As the speed increases, you can expect to see a slow, steady increase in lactate until eventually there will be a sharp rise in the line on the graph, indicating that your blood levels have crossed the threshold and are not being eliminated thoroughly. By training close to your threshold (but not exceeding it), you can help maximize your run improvements.

In conclusion

Baseline measures should be an essential component of your running program. Without obtaining a baseline you will not be able to effectively monitor whether you as a runner are making any improvements in either your run-specific or health-specific factors. Consequently, you will not be able to determine whether your current running plan is having a positive effect. Baseline values should be captured as soon after starting your running program as possible; however, if you have already started then you should obtain baseline measures immediately. The choice as to what measures to obtain are up to you and should be matched with your intended running goals – if you are aiming to improve your running ability, focus on aerobic capacity or lactate threshold. Health-related goals such as an intent to lose weight should center around obtaining baseline values of fat mass or cholesterol level. Regardless of your ultimate goal with running, baseline values serve to provide valuable feedback as to your progress towards that goal.

Chapter 4: Use the right running equipment

One of the beautiful things about running is that its participation costs are minimal compared to that of other sports. You don't need a specific facility, or required protective equipment, or outlandish technology to go for a run, and you can usually start your run right outside of your front door. This gives you as a runner the ability to run when you want and where you want – a freedom not offered by many other sporting activities.

Although there is no real requirement for running equipment, it is important to understand that maximizing your success with running does require at least a minimum investment in some key items that will benefit you on your runs. In this chapter we will cover several of those items, and I will attempt to group these items into *essential* versus *recommended* equipment. By making a relatively small financial commitment to a few key items, your running can be more comfortable, more efficient, and less likely to invite injury.

Before we get into a discussion of running equipment, understand that this chapter is designed to provide you an overview of your options. It is by no means intended to imply that you *need* these items. Our bodies are designed to run already – it doesn't know the latest technology or perform only when wearing the most shock-absorbing shoes. Therefore, we will explore the various equipment so as to make you a more informed runner and potentially make you more comfortable in the process. There is a wealth of running gear out there, and we will not discuss every possible option. Hats, ear-warmers, gloves, and other ancillary items don't have as much direct effect on your runs and so won't be discussed here.

Essential equipment

Shoes

I can make no stronger recommendation for an investment in running equipment than I will for a quality pair of running shoes. Shoes are what allow you to run the way you do and are involved in every aspect of your run.

A lot can be said about shoes, largely because they factor so much into running. Running shoes come in all shapes, sizes, and prices. You can easily find running shoes for under $30 all the way up to high-end running shoes that approach the $200 range.

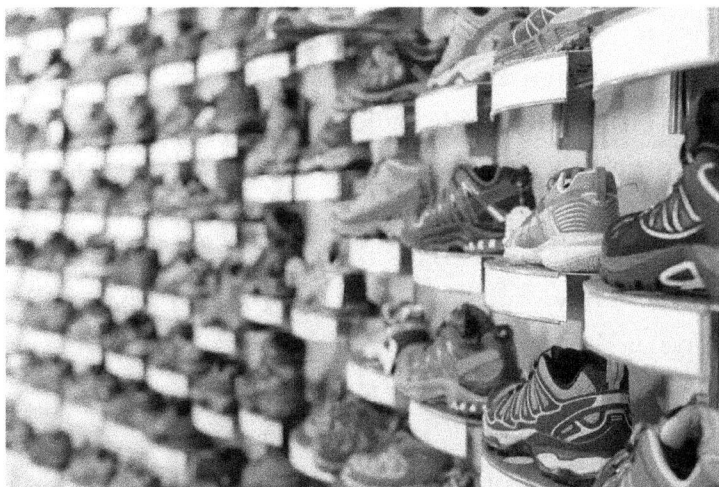

Given the vast amount of options available when it comes to running shoes, you should be able to find the style you want at a price you can afford without having to compromise on quality.

Regardless of your price range, the key issue lies in finding shoes that are comfortable *for you*. Don't rely on what your friends recommend, or what brand you see most often at a race. Because feet are so different from person-to-person, it is imperative that you find shoes that both match your anatomy and meet your specific preferences for comfort and style.

Gait analysis

Somewhat related to your anatomy as well as the shoes you wear is what is known as your *gait*. Gait is effectively the specific leg movement pattern that a person uses when running. Your stride length, foot strike, hip motion, knee extension, and other factors all comprise your gait, and no two people have exactly the same gait. Because your gait is also related to how your foot strikes the ground, it is important that you have your gait analyzed to see if a particular type of shoe can help reduce your risk of injury and positively influence your stride.

Gait analysis can be highly or minimally involved depending on the training of the person analyzing your gait as well as the type of equipment used. In terms of equipment, I've seen everything from a video camera in a sporting goods store to a biomechanical image capture system used for gait analysis, operated by anyone from a store employee to a PhD-level biomechanist. The level of analysis you can get is a personal preference, and you will find a wide variety in price differences – from free to $100 or more for a highly technical analysis.

The purpose of a gait analysis is to evaluate your gait and match any potential problems to a specific shoe. For example, some people *over-pronate* when they run, meaning that when their foot hits the ground it is "rolled inward" too far. This changes the mechanics of how their foot is designed to work, and can arguably cost that individual in terms of running efficiency. Recognizing such an issue during a gait analysis can help match that individual with a shoe designed to correct over-pronation and potentially reduce their risk of future injury. Similarly, under-pronation may exist, or it may be revealed that the runner has a neutral running gait, which typically does not require a corrective shoe and in turn opens that individual to more shoe choices.

Understand that gait analysis is not required, and if you avoid it you will not likely suffer some preventable running injury. Rather, gait analysis is effective at improving your running efficiency and correcting any potential gait abnormalities. These factors are extremely important for competitive runners but may not be much of a priority for someone just starting out or running only occasionally. Still, given that you can get a gait analysis for free at many locations, I highly recommend that you do so.

Shock absorption

If you are running for the health benefits, I would venture to guess that you don't run to get injured but instead to prevent long-term health conditions that come in the form of heart disease, weight gain, etc. In some cases, however, a cheap shoe can actually increase your risk of injury which can in turn knock you out of running for an extended period of time. The repetitive pounding that parts of your lower body take during a run can be damaging without proper protection. However, you can help limit the amount of force transmitted to your lower body with a quality pair of shoes that provides ample cushioning.

Cushioning should factor in to the overall comfort of a shoe. Again, be sure to avoid the temptation of taking into account what another runner may recommend when it comes to a shoe's cushioning or comfort. Why? Because as we discussed earlier, different people have different running gaits. Your running partner may have a heel-strike running gait, requiring adequate cushioning in the heel. You may instead be a midfoot runner, meaning that your running gait places the majority of landing force on the ball of your foot. Different shoes have different cushioning design, and you should match a particular shoe with your own running gait. If you are a midfoot runner, because your heel is not a primary shock absorber there is not necessarily a priority on finding a shoe that emphasizes cushioning in the heel. Furthermore, understand that when it comes to shock absorption, it may take a week of running or more to determine whether a shoe is a particularly good fit for you.

Comfort

Selecting a shoe based on overall comfort is extremely important, and should go hand-in-hand with shock absorption. If you skimp on comfort, allowing a slightly uncomfortable shoe in favor of a lighter or more fashionable shoe, I'm almost certain that you'll regret it in the long run and will not be fully enjoying your runs. And even the most comfortable shoe may not ultimately work out for you, either. The most comfortable running shoe I have ever worn lasted me just a few miles. Despite feeling like a firm pillow around my feet, the shoe quickly wore a blister on both my left and right arches. So, comfort in that case was over-ruled by an injury factor that would significantly affect my running ability. Particularly frustrating was that the shoe was recommended by almost everyone in my running group, light in weight, and had great shock absorption. I ended up getting a different pair and was happy with them, but they didn't have the amazing comfort level of the initial pair.

Weight

Besides comfort, one of the most important factors that I personally look for in a running shoe is weight. Go down a row of shoes and you will find that weight can vary significantly even between running shoes. Most sporting goods stores will include the shoe's weight on the price sticker, suggesting to me that weight is becoming a more popular consideration in the shoe-buying process.

Weight is important simply because the weight of a shoe influences how hard your legs have to work. More weight makes the legs work harder, in turn causing more energy to be burned in addition to potentially increasing the risk for muscle injury. Because of the extra weight which in turn requires a slight bit more energy to move, a heavier shoe can cause you to fatigue faster. Shoes are typically weighed in ounces, and even an ounce can add up.

For example, if you run a race with 5000 steps for each leg, and you chose a shoe weighing one ounce more than your second choice, each leg has to provide energy to move an extra 316 pounds over the course of the race, or the total amount of energy required to move one ounce 5000 times. Therefore, your body has to supply energy to perform an extra 632 pounds of work, as both legs must do the work. Double that amount for a shoe that is two ounces heavier than you need, quadruple it for a shoe four ounces heavier, and so on. Furthermore, as your run distance increases, the subsequent energy requirement increases proportionally for even small differences in shoe weight. As you can see, even very small weight differences can add up.

Clearly, shoe weight can make a difference. However, you don't want to have the mindset that the lighter a shoe, the better. There will be a certain point at which weight will compromise structure, and that can be detrimental to your runs over time. For example, to get to a certain weight a shoe design may need to reduce padding, or have a lower collar, or a thinner tongue. These can affect aspects of the shoe such as shock absorption, or can cause a painful blister if the shoe rubs you in just the right place. Similarly, don't compromise on comfort or fit in favor of a lighter shoe. If a shoe is not comfortable during your run, I would suspect that the consequences are worse than any energy savings made by going with a slightly lighter shoe. Therefore, factor shoe weight in only after you have first narrowed down your choices to a group of running shoes based on fit and comfort. Then consider a shoe that offers light weight in conjunction with fit and comfort.

Styles

You are going to notice that there are a lot of different styles of shoes out there. Cross-training, running, trail, and minimalist are each a type of shoe with a relatively specific purpose. For what you will be doing – running – you will be best served to purchase a running shoe. The other shoes will work to some degree, but they have different design elements such as a wider base or minimal shock-absorption that could serve to negatively affect your runs for a variety of reasons. Therefore, I recommend that you start out with a good pair of running shoes initially, and then experiment with other shoes as necessary.

Don't expect to find one shoe type and stick with it for years. Shoe companies generally change their model or style yearly, so even though you may find the perfect look or perfect fit, that same shoe design may well be gone within six to 12 months. Therefore, if you are absolutely sold on a particular shoe – great! You have found the Holy Grail of shoe compatibility that others only dream of finding. If this occurs, the smart thing to do would be to buy a couple pairs and keep them in your closet until your initial pair needs replacing. Doing this will help ensure that you have an ample supply of an identical running shoe for the foreseeable future.

One caveat to finding that 'perfect' shoe is that it can take you awhile to get to a point where you know which shoe is best. That usually comes through years of running, buying shoes that fit great and buying shoes that you almost instantly regret. My point is that just because you have a new shoe that feels great, it doesn't mean that it's necessarily the perfect shoe. You will want to pay attention to tread wear, fabric breathability, and overall shoe quality over time as well. Gradually, you will begin to notice a particular shoe that holds up better than previous models due to a higher quality of design. That model will ultimately become your preferred shoe.

Price

Price is not what I would consider a characteristic of a shoe, but unfortunately it's often what people pay the most attention to. I would venture to say that price should be the *least* important aspect of a shoe that you factor into a purchasing decision. Unfortunately, price is often established more on marketing or advertising than on quality, meaning that name brand shoes may cost more simply because of the brand and not because of any high-tech design features. Still, consumers can get sucked in by crafty marketing and pay unnecessarily high prices for a shoe just as easily as they can choose to avoid a quality lower-priced shoe simply because it's not a name brand.

Go to any sporting goods store and you will find an array of running shoes. If in the market for a new pair of running shoes, you will want to spend a good amount of time trying on those shoes you are interested in. Try a few on that are below your price point as well as a few that are above. Avoid the mindset that expensive shoes are good and inexpensive shoes are bad, and avoid focusing initially on a shoe that appears fashionable. As I mentioned earlier, the most comfortable pair of running shoes I have *ever* worn caused large blisters on both of my arches within the first few miles of a run, and these shoes were relatively expensive at $130. Despite their high price and comfort, they just couldn't work for me and I ultimately had to take them back and get a different pair. So again, don't focus on price and don't assume that expense influences how well the shoe will work for you.

During the initial stages of finding a good pair of shoes, remember that you are striving to narrow your choice down to a few shoes that fit your feet best as well as meet your standards for the other shoe qualifications that we have discussed. Therefore, ignore shoe price in the early decision stages. In a perfect world, you will end up with a variety of shoes that meet your standards, at which point you could then factor in price and aesthetic quality. Most likely, you will and should end up conceding on at least one preferred characteristic (e.g. color, price, etc.) in favor of a quality fit and comfort.

Shoe Replacement

We've talked at length about shoes, but as we all know, even the best running shoes will need replacement eventually. What do you want to look for to know it's time to replace your running shoes? This can be a time of excitement or dread for a runner, depending on whether the thought of new shoes is viewed as a chance to improve one's running or if it instead means having to fork over what may be a significant amount of cash for a new pair. Regardless, you have to accept that your running shoes are going to wear out. One favorable way to look at the situation is to recognize that if your shoes are indeed wearing out, it signifies that you are likely maintaining a pretty significant amount of running activity.

Running shoes should not be viewed like that roll of toothpaste in your bathroom – don't try to squeeze every last possible ounce of use out of them. Part of the problem is that you are most likely basing your shoe replacement decision on visual aspects such as how much tread remains. Depending on the type of surface that you run on, tread may or may not wear faster than the supportive aspects of the shoe. For example, if you run on hard jagged asphalt you will likely wear out your tread much faster than the shock-absorbing aspects of the shoe. Therefore, while it may look as though the shoe is 'old' due to reduced tread, the shoe may in fact still be well within its useful life. Conversely, if you run on soft surfaces such as grass or rubber, your shoe may show very little tread wear despite significant failure of structural components.

Rather than wait for some visual aspect of your shoe to indicate that it's time for replacement, it is often recommended that you replace the shoe while it still has some useful qualities remaining. If you don't, you'll likely be running in a shoe that has little protective cushioning or arch support, thereby increasing your risk for certain injuries. Most runners and professionals will tell you that after 500 miles of use you should replace your shoes with a new pair. Others suggest that shoe technology has advanced enough to allow continued use of your shoe into the 600-700 mile range, so again, the final choice is ultimately left up to you.

Data Collection Devices

This topic could easily be titled "GPS Trackers" or even "watches", as they both are useful in collecting data. The difference though is in the type and amount of data collected. For you, it is important to ensure that you are monitoring several run factors in order to compare yourself over time, which we talked about in a previous chapter. But for now, we'll look at a few different data collection devices that you can use to help improve your running.

Digital Watch

The most basic of data collection devices is the simple digital watch. Digital watches traditionally tell you the time and date, but the right type can also provide a stopwatch and in many cases a countdown timer. Although this rather basic amount of run data (e.g. total time) is not necessarily as beneficial for an experienced runner, digital watches provide enough data to get newer runners started and do allow you to track and evaluate your run progress over time.

One of the main functions of a digital watch will be to record your total running time. Start the watch when you begin running, and stop it when you finish. The time between those two points is your total run time. If you know your distance, you can divide the distance by your time to get your *pace.* When calculated by your run time and distance, your pace – usually reported in minutes-per-mile – provides an overall average pace of your run. However, this pace is estimated based on your overall time – it is not specific to any particular portion of your run. Consequently, if you stopped at a traffic light for 20 seconds or sprinted the last quarter mile of your run, those variables won't be observable in the 'total time ran'. Furthermore, as a digital watch only records time, it is difficult to determine your pace while you are running, unless you know specific mile markers and can record and calculate the time it takes to run the distance between those markers.

Your digital watch may also have a countdown timer. Timers are effective for challenging yourself when attempting to run a certain distance in a certain time. By seeing the actual time remaining, some people can be motivated to increase their running pace in order to beat the timer.

GPS Tracking

While digital watches provide data relevant to running time and overall pace, more advanced technology such as Global Positioning System (GPS) devices can report much more data. For example, they can report your real-time pace at any point during your run. Similarly, they can provide a constant real-time measure of how far you have run up to your current location. Several styles work in conjunction with a heart rate monitor to record your heart rate while running. Each of these variables can provide you valuable feedback during a run.

Price range for GPS watches is dependent upon the features you choose. The minimally equipped watches will track your distance covered over the day by measuring your steps, while the top-of-the-line watches measure heart rate, speed, and distance, and can also monitor other sport activities such as triathlon-related swimming and biking. With various options you will also find that price increases proportionally, so expect to spend from $100 for a minimal-feature watch up to and exceeding $600 or more for a multi-sport watch.

An important factor that makes some of the higher-end GPS watches so attractive is that you can download your running information (e.g. pace, distance, heart rate, etc.) onto a computer or app in order to look at trends over time. For example, if you buy your watch when you first start out running, you can track how your run distance improves, or perhaps how your run completion time decreases from week to week. Or, you may want to evaluate your heart rate over time to determine what zone you are achieving while running. The programs that these GPS watches come can be quite extensive, and what you do with the program can be dependent upon how much effort you want to spend looking at and interpreting your data. But as we discussed in the previous chapter, tracking your data over time can be a great motivator and allows you to determine whether your workouts are having a beneficial effect.

Clothing

Run clothing is one of those items that you don't necessarily have to buy, but you will enjoy your run more if you do. You can certainly take any old t-shirt out of your closet as well as a pair of mesh shorts and throw on some cotton socks and still have a great run. With a lot of the traditional cotton clothing, though, your sweat tends to absorb into the clothing, making it heavier and more likely to drag against your skin. I learned this lesson fiercely one time when running in a t-shirt and basketball shorts as a rainstorm started. I was about two miles away from my starting point and had to traverse that return distance in a full-on downpour. In less than a minute the shorts were soaked and flopping back and forth across my legs, so much so that I had to reach down and hold them still. Meanwhile my shirt became severely weighted down as it became saturated with water. As I continued to run back towards my starting point, not only did the shorts annoy me endlessly but the cotton shirt bouncing up and down in time with my pace ended up murdering my nipples. The next day I bought my first true run-type clothing, and to this day I have never again ran in traditional cotton shirts or non-running shorts.

The newer styles of running clothes are designed to be breathable, meaning that they have a better ability to allow air to pass through the fibers, in turn carrying some moisture with the moving air. However, most traditional cotton clothing fibers tend to retain moisture within the fibers. Moisture-wicking clothing is typically made of polyester blends, which have a difficult time holding on to moisture and as such retain much less of that moisture in their fibers than found with cotton clothing. In addition, these polyester fibers are often treated chemically so as to further reduce their ability to hold moisture within the fibers. And, while cotton might be more naturally breathable (but also more apt to hold moisture) than polyester, manufacturers can weave the polyester fibers to allow microscopic 'channels' to help move moisture out to where it can be readily evaporated.

Now that both running shirts and shorts come in polyester fabric, you will have a wealth of run clothing options to choose from. Functionality is probably a little less important here than with shoes, but you will still want a light, breathable, and sweat-wicking option for running, and even more so if you are running in hot weather. Furthermore, you will find two predominant options when it comes to run clothing – loose-fitting and compression style. Compression shirts and shorts are typically made of lycra, polyester, nylon, or spandex. The theories behind the benefits of compression gear vary, with some arguments suggesting that compression gear aids in recovery and/or blood flow, while others counter that any effect is "all in your head". Regardless, there are generally no real running detriments to wearing compression gear, so it is generally left up to you as a personal preference.

Alongside compression gear you will find the lighter loose-fitting running shirts and shorts. True running shorts (as compared to say 'basketball shorts') are made of lightweight synthetic material such as polyester, nylon, or a polyester-spandex blend. Running shorts can also be found in cotton or wool, yet as you now know the moisture-wicking capability of these fibers is reduced and can result in cotton or wool-type shorts retaining more moisture (and thereby increasing one's risk of chafing). Running shorts can be found with or without pockets to hold various items such as a key or identification. And many running shorts include a built-in liner to provide support, which depending on the runner may allow the runner to forego the need to wear underwear or compression shorts.

Because of the wide success of wicking technology, almost all run clothing has polyester options. Even socks have been brought into the discussion about the benefits of polyester, though they can still be found in cotton as well. There's not a whole lot of unique technology in socks when it comes to running, though you may have personal preferences as to whether you want low-cut, high, or some other length of sock. And, some socks have been designed to have additional features such as an arch support sewn into the sock itself which may be preferable to your own running style.

In addition to what we have discussed, there is a wide variety of specialized accessory clothing options available for runners. Sports bras, compression shorts, headbands, and compression sleeves are just a few of the options available to help you maximize the effects of your run. These items come from a wide variety of manufacturers and can therefore be found in a variety of colors, styles, and prices. Like most all items you can purchase, you will likely get what you pay for when it comes to quality and durability. Furthermore, spend time online doing your research to see if the product is worthwhile or perhaps just a passing fad. Outside of the scientific literature, my favorite research is to read as many online reviews of a particular product as I can. The relatively unfiltered responses you can read reveal much about a product, and if you take the time

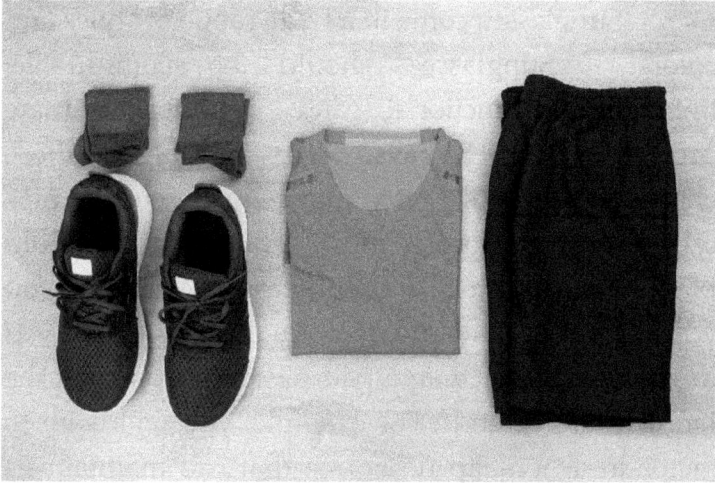

Despite a wealth of available running accessories, essential run clothing should include shoes, socks, a shirt, and shorts designed for running.

to wade through the ineffective reviews that complain about things like 'the shipping box was damaged', you can gain some valuable information about a product.

Sunglasses

Running is generally an outdoor sport, so it should be expected that you will be exposed to the sun quite often. While you may choose a hat or visor to help provide some eye protection from the sun, a good pair of sunglasses can go a long way toward protecting your eyes from the brightness of the sun as well as ultraviolet (UV) rays.

Sunglasses come in a wide range of styles and colors. Sunglasses should be comfortable, lightweight, functional, and provide adequate protection from UV rays. After checking off those characteristics, it's pretty much up to you to pick which style you prefer most. Functionality should play an important role in sunglass selection, as you will want a pair that holds up to the rigors involved in running rather than a pair designed based on the latest fashion trend. For example, you will want to factor in a non-slip nosepiece that can maintain its function when you are sweaty, as well as lenses that limit fogging as your body temperature or the air temperature changes. Similarly, sunglasses that rest right up against your eyebrows may collect sweat that eventually drips down through the middle of the lens, thereby clouding your vision. It is tough to clean your lenses when you are soaked in sweat, so again, functionality is important.

Like shoes, sunglasses come in a wide range of prices, styles, and function. I recommend that you try on several different pair in order to establish what works for you, but also be aware that you probably won't truly know the functionality of a pair of sunglasses until you're out on a run. Regardless, finding a good pair of quality sunglasses can be extremely beneficial for helping you enjoy your runs.

In conclusion

Having quality equipment can go a long way in helping you enjoy your runs. While you can certainly start running at almost no additional cost, investing in at least a good pair of shoes can have significant dividends for you in the long run. Furthermore, considering a set of polyester-type clothing to wear during your runs can help keep you cool and comfortable during those summer months when the sun and heat can be ruthless. Because quality equipment can not only make your runs more enjoyable but also improve your running outcomes, I recommend that you strongly consider the benefits of investing in a good set of running gear.

Chapter 5: Find a quality route

One of the benefits to running outdoors is that you get to experience nature – the sun, the breeze, perhaps the cool air, or any of the other elements at that particular time of the year. With indoor running, you might have a fan blowing air on you, the air conditioner keeping the house cool, or perhaps a television to watch, but you don't have access to the scenery, breeze, and variability that often comes with outdoor running. Though some may prefer indoor running for the above-mentioned factors, many prefer to run outdoor when available. In doing so, the calm, controlled environment inherent to indoor running is not available, and you are often left to the fate dealt you in the way of traffic, running surfaces, or even weather. This is, of course, assuming that you have an adequate place to run outdoors, which may not always be the case in the event that you live in a big city or perhaps even out in the country.

Availability

For most of us, we will have some level of access to a relatively flat, stable (i.e. solid) surface of enough distance that allows us to complete a respectable run. Your route may be a sidewalk, street, road, high school track, or even parking lot, but having a safe and stable surface is imperative for both your own safety as well as in reducing the risk of injury.

One limiting factor for outdoor running is the requirement that you have a place to run. Most all sporting activities require some sort of venue to occur. Sports such as basketball require a very flat, hard surface as well as boundary markers and a proper goal. Swimming requires a pool or lake with adequate water temperatures. Running might be considered the least problematic when it comes to finding an adequate venue, as you can literally walk out your front door to start running. For many of us, our runs will involve a sidewalk or street. Others may have a gravel road. Regardless of what you have available, if it is designed for foot traffic or a vehicle it can serve as an adequate running surface assuming that you are cognizant of potential traffic concerns or other safety issues (i.e. uneven surfaces, potholes, etc.).

Most runners can find a sidewalk or other appropriate surface to run on without issue. However, if you live in a large city, there may be a stoplight at every block, or tree roots pushing whole sections of sidewalk up out of the ground that make for a very unstable running surface. Similarly, an individual living in a rural environment may live on a dirt road that becomes muddy with even the lightest rain. Such conditions can severely limit the quality of your run and must be accounted for when determining your running route. If you live in an area with poor sidewalks or traffic congestion, you may be better off driving somewhere to get in a decent run. Or, a hard rain may render your route impassible for two, three, or more days. In such cases, it is important to establish a contingency plan that will still allow you to run when your primary route is unavailable.

Safety

One of the most important aspects of the route you take is your overall safety. Fully enclosed areas such as a high school running track or running path can help you avoid dangerous vehicle traffic while running outdoors, and if you have close access to such a venue it can be a great asset for your running. Furthermore, the surface at most school running tracks is impeccable as it is designed for running, and can thereby reduce your risk for injury.

For those of us without easy access to a running track or path, city streets and sidewalks often

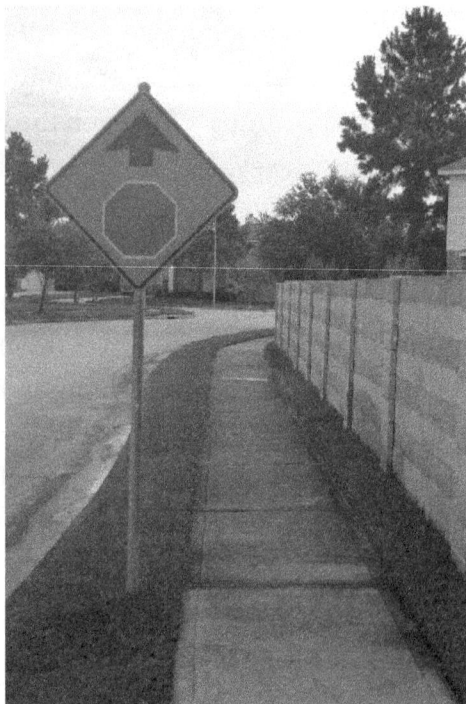

Although sidewalks provide a safe route away from traffic, they do not come without their own safety hazards. Here, a metal street sign hangs over the sidewalk, which can cause a significant injury if a runner is not mindful of his or her surroundings.

provide the next-best option. Sidewalks allow a relative amount of safety from vehicle traffic as they lie separate from the road. However, sidewalks also come with their own set of risks to runners that may not be immediately considered. For example, the running surface of a sidewalk is not always ideal. Individual sidewalk sections can separate due to shifting or an underlying tree root which can create raised sidewalk edges of an inch or more. Such raised areas can be a major tripping risk to runners. Low-hanging tree branches, gate drains, toys and other items, or even other runners can increase the injury risk when running on sidewalks. You should decide if the risk is acceptable to you and factor that decision in with the individual laws of your state or city regarding running in the street versus the sidewalk.

Another issue with sidewalk running involves what can happen as you approach an intersection. It is important to note whether the intersection is a four-way stop, two-way stop, or if traffic does not stop. If traffic does not stop at the intersection, runners must be aware that they will need to stop well-prior to reaching the street in order to prevent evasive action by an oncoming car. Even if approaching a two-way or four-way stop, runners must ensure that the driver sees them. Drivers arriving at a four-way stop typically focus their eyes on the road to look for approaching cars rather than on a sidewalk.

Even though pedestrians have the right of way at an intersection, runners must take caution to ensure that drivers see them before passing through. The driver could be looking for cars, or the runner could be in line with the windshield pillar (the metal bars on each side of a windshield) which would effectively 'hide' the runner from the driver's view,

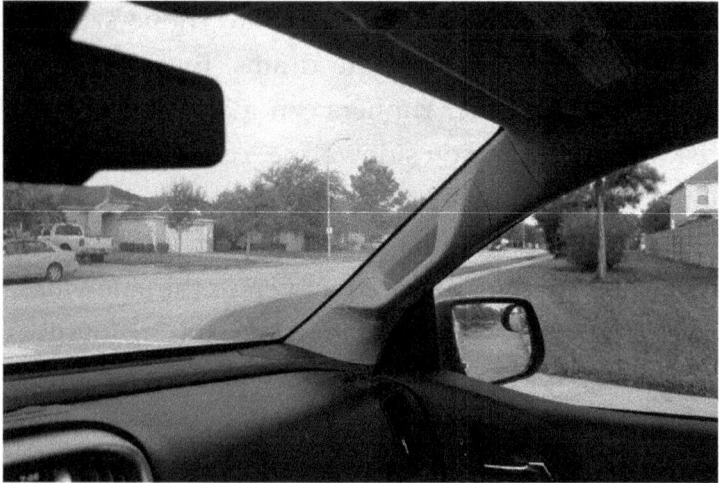

Notice how when stopped at an intersection the windshield pillar can effectively block the driver's view of a runner approaching on the sidewalk.

particularly if a driver is planning to make a right turn and slightly turns to the right before coming to a complete stop. Stopped cars making this slight turn can end up positioning the windshield pillar directly in line with the sidewalk, further obstructing any runner who might be approaching the intersection from a sidewalk on the passenger side of the car.

If sidewalks are not available, runners may be relegated to run in the road. This is particularly dangerous and should be avoided at all costs. In fact, if a sidewalk exists most states and local municipalities have laws in place that *require* the runner to use the sidewalk. If that is the case, you must follow the individual law governing the particular area (county, city, state, etc.) that you are in, as you might have little legal standing if you as a runner are in an accident that results from not following the local sidewalk-use requirements.

When there is any interaction with a road during their runs, runners must recognize that they are expected to adhere to all roadway regulations. For example, runners should not cross a controlled (e.g. traffic light) intersection when stopped for a red light, and should not enter the road if the stoplight has already turned yellow. Furthermore, runners should only cross an intersection when they receive a "Walk" signal. Yes, your pace or expected finishing time will be interrupted if you encounter a "Don't Walk" sign, but safety should always take precedence over convenience. Furthermore, you could be risking your own legal liability as a result of not adhering to traffic laws. Because of the vast array of regulations and devices that can be found at intersections, runners should make themselves familiar with all local and state regulations regarding pedestrians.

There are of course situations where the sidewalk is either under repair or non-existent and the runner must run on a road or street. In these cases, it is imperative that the runner wear highly-visible clothing – including reflective material if running in low-light conditions – in order to allow drivers the best opportunity to see him or her. In those situations where sidewalks are not available, it is almost always recommended in the United States that the runner use the side of the road that faces traffic. This is to help ensure that he or she can see the activity of oncoming traffic, and allows time for the runner to avert oncoming danger if necessary. However, be aware that in many states, if a sidewalk is available, the runner must use the sidewalk or face legal consequences if running in the road. Again, it is up to the runner to be familiar with his or her state and local regulations.

Runners must also be aware that even though they run on a sidewalk, they may be forced into the street at some point. At certain intersections, sidewalks may angle toward a main street so that if a runner does not alter their pace, he or she may inadvertently run out into the road.

Similarly, running on a sidewalk in a residential area will often find the runner encountering sidewalks blocked by cars that are

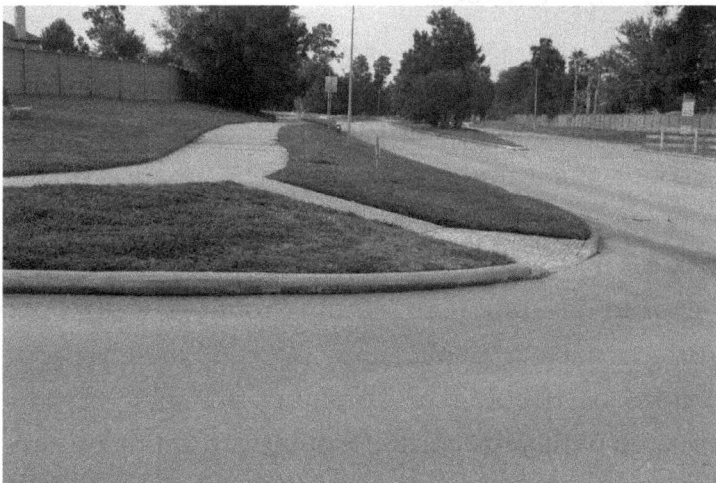

Sidewalk design may set up the possibility that a runner's momentum could carry him or her into the roadway, as demonstrated by this downhill sidewalk.

parked in the driveway. In actuality, blocking a sidewalk is generally illegal for this very reason – it forces individuals into the street where the risk of being struck by a car is heightened. Even if the car belongs to the homeowner, the pathway formed by the sidewalk should be unimpeded, even across an individual's driveway. If you encounter a blocked

91

sidewalk, you should use caution in maneuvering around the offending car and ensure that you check for traffic prior to reaching the blocked area in the event that you would need to enter the road.

Running surface

Once you have accounted for safety by finding an adequate location or route, you need to take into account the running surface. The quality of the running surface can play a role in influencing your risk for injury and should at least be considered as a factor in deciding your running route as well. Poor surfaces such as an old sidewalk could increase your chance of tripping or spraining an ankle if it is covered with large cracks. Similarly, running on very loose gravel or sand can significantly increase the amount of effort needed to run, thereby reducing your pace and potentially the amount of total distance you are able to cover.

When sidewalks are your running route of choice, it is best to scout out a route that keeps you on the smoothest possible surface. For example, tree roots can often displaced sidewalk sections and can in turn present a significant hazard to runners. Even a ¼″ protrusion up into the running surface can set up the possibility of tripping, so it is important to remain cognizant of running surface fluctuations. In addition, sidewalks often end at curbed intersections, thereby requiring the runner to step down 8-10 inches onto the street as well as stepping back up again onto the next sidewalk. All of these situations can invite the opportunity for a lower-limb injury such as a rolled ankle; therefore, runners should try to plan the safest route and avoid distractions during your run that may take your gaze away from the oncoming sidewalk surface.

Unpaved surfaces

Non-paved surfaces work well for running, too. In fact, softer surfaces such as dirt or grass are often recommended as a running surface due to the reduction in stress that is applied to the lower leg. Whether it's a dirt road or the increasingly popular trail-running type of venue, non-paved surfaces offer a unique experience for runners. If non-paved running is an option for you, you may wish to consider a switch to a shoe designed especially for off-road running. Trail shoes tend to have a thicker tread pattern, less cushioning, and are lower to the ground than traditional hard-surface running shoes. These modifications are due to the more unstable yet softer surfaces associated with trail running compared to that of road running.

When it comes to trails, be aware that the running surface can vary widely. Small holes, roots, loose sand, or small rocks are common on trails and you must be diligent in monitoring the running surface constantly when trail running. Most trails receive minimal manicuring, as they may proceed through forests or across rocky terrain. Therefore, be aware of the potential for lower-limb injuries on trails, as well as the potential for delayed care if the trail or unpaved road is somewhat isolated. Because of the extended time frame that may result if you are injured while trail running, ensure that you always have at minimum a signaling device and/or cell phone with you when trail running.

Familiar vs Unfamiliar

Depending on where you live you may or may not have a lot of different options for which route you take. If running on a non-paved surface, for example, you may only have one option for a running route, as alternative routes may have the presence of erosion, or mud, or may not provide a consistent, stable surface. Conversely, interconnected paved roads and sidewalks such as can be found in the city may allow you significantly more options regarding which route to take. As a runner, having options will definitely work in your favor.

My preferred route of running occurs along wide, suburban streets and sidewalks with relatively little traffic outside of morning and afternoon rush hours. Typically my runs occur between 5-6am when traffic is not a real concern. For me, the opportunities as to which direction to run are endless given the amount of open roads in the area. Nevertheless, over time I developed a preferred route that offers wide sidewalks, minimal intersections, and relatively scenic views. My familiarity with this route also allows me to establish where I am at distance-wise during any particular point of my run, as mile markers and even half-mile markers become easily recognized after many trips using my GPS watch.

Types of Routes

When you plan your day's running route, there are three predominant options available. Which type of route you choose is largely up to you, but may be influenced somewhat by the terrain, your available time, or in some cases even weather. And as we will discuss, there are positive and negative aspects of each type of route available to you.

Out-and-back

Routes that take the same path out as they do on the return are known as out-and-back courses. If your route requires you to run a particular distance, turn around, and then run that same distance back, you are on an out-and-back course. Such a course requires only half of the amount of running path compared to other types of routes since you are running over the same route in each direction.

Personally, the out-and-back route is my favorite for the same reason that others may see an out-and-back as a detriment – it forces you to run at least twice as far as the point at which you turn around. If, for example, I am on a six mile run (three miles 'there and back'), if I feel an onset of fatigue at mile two I still have to run at least an additional two miles to get back to the start, which is usually my house. This in effect 'forces' me to run at least a minimal distance, with that distance being twice the distance at which I reach a turnaround point. With other route types I may be on a loop and can easily cut my run short at any point that I pass by my house.

Another benefit of the out-and-back is that if you have a headwind on the out trip, the reverse leg will provide a tailwind. This is actually something I plan for, as I prefer to have a headwind on the *out* portion given that I will be more tired on the return phase and would prefer the assistance of a tailwind. Others may feel that a headwind on the return phase is preferred as it can have more of a cooling effect on the body due to the increased airflow across the body. As with many running-related choices, your own preference may differ.

Along these same lines, a negative of the out-and-back is that if you *must* stop your run, you are a significant distance away from the start and must still get back somehow. This could be a problem if you suffer an injury at mile three of a six mile out-and-back, or if a storm develops suddenly. If that happened, you would still have at least a three-mile trek back to the start, which could be problematic in some certain situations. Separately, some feel that a negative of the return trip of an out-and-back is that you are seeing the same scenery which can make that particular portion of the run seem a bit longer and somewhat monotonous. This can actually be turned into a positive though, as a return trip on the same route allows you to know what to expect during the second half of your run. Should you enter a running event such as a half marathon, you may find that certain courses actually *repeat* an out-and-back one or more times.

Loops

A loop is quite simply a run that requires several turns along the route that results in you returning automatically to the starting point. A run around a city block would be a loop run, as would a run around several city blocks. Most park trails are some form of a loop, allowing you to start your run and pass that starting position one or more times depending on the length of your run.

Loop courses have the benefit that all scenery along the loop will be new throughout the entire loop as there is no 'return portion' like there is on an out-and-back. However, because you are returning to the original start position, any downhill slope that you encounter during the course will assuredly be followed by an uphill portion, as any gain or loss in elevation must be neutralized by the end of your loop. Another component of loop running that could be viewed as a potential positive *or* negative is that every loop has a 'point of no return' such that if you are injured, experience unfavorable weather, or fatigue early it may be a shorter distance to actually complete the loop than to turn around and head back. In addition, if you plan to pass any services such as a bathroom or drinking fountain, loop runs may only allow it to occur once per loop, while out-and-back runs will likely result in at least two passes.

Point-to-Point

If you have ever wanted to just run and not worry about the route you take, a point-to-point is probably what you had in mind. With point-to-point runs, you do not end at the same place you start. Say you want to head down some deserted road as far as you can go. If you have set up a means to get a ride back to your starting point, you would be making a point-to-point run. Such runs offer quite a bit of freedom, even allowing you to plan out your route during the run itself as you have no concerns about ensuring that you return in a timely fashion to your starting point.

Like loop runs, point-to-point routes provide all new scenery, and you only have to experience each portion once since there is no return portion. However, if your route takes you directly into a headwind (or tailwind), you might have that headwind the *entire* portion of the run. Similarly, with a well-thought-out course you could even have a downhill run the entire distance of your route.

The biggest negative of a point-to-point run is that it will typically require a form of transportation back to your starting point. Therefore, point-to-points are not a common route when going out for a simple run on your own.

Matching your route to your goal

No matter if you're running just to run or you're preparing for a running event, you will almost always have some sort of outcome that you are working towards. As such, you should be mindful of what you are wanting to accomplish when you plan out your route. Always, always match your training to your goals and design your training runs to best help you accomplish your goals.

If, for example, you have been completing training runs for the past couple of weeks, you may be interested in seeing if you can set a new personal record for covering a particular distance in the shortest amount of time. If so, I would recommend planning out the flattest course with the fewest interruptions. Therefore, try to design a route that avoids stoplights as well as other potential conflicts that might slow you down. If you choose a route that includes hills, the extra effort required may cause you to have a slower time, in turn making it appear as though you have made no improvement when in fact your improvement was actually countered by the additional effort required to maneuver the hills.

Separately, you may have times that you would prefer to plan a route that has hills. This is especially relevant if you are entering a race that encounters hills, as training only on a flat surface prior to the race would make for a very frustrating time on race day. In the fitness world, this practice of matching your training with your goals is known as *specificity*. I have many routes in my suburban neighborhoods that have hilly, somewhat aesthetic sidewalks right alongside very flat roads. To avoid the up-and-down nature of the sidewalk path I often prefer to utilize the flatter road for my own running. Other runners might prefer to incorporate hill running into their workouts to build endurance and provide a bit of strength work, or to better prepare them for a hilly race.

Internet-based route planning

No matter where you live or travel, I would bet that you can find a pre-designed route near you that someone else has put up on the internet. Given the wide range of running apps and websites, there are a vast amount of options available to help you search for a pre-planned route to use when running, especially when you are in unfamiliar territory. Furthermore, you can tailor your search results by distance, location, and even running surface to help match you up with the type of route that you intend to take on. Many of these routes include comments from the original designer that may alert you to particular concerns such as traffic issues or road surface conditions.

Another helpful option is that you can plan out any distance right from your computer. Twenty years ago you were stuck 'guesstimating' the distance of a planned route or just running the route itself in order to determine the actual running distance. These days, computer maps allow you to plot out turn-by-turn directions, then automatically calculate the total distance of your planned route whether it is an out-and-back or a loop course. Unfortunately, planning out a route from scratch on the computer doesn't account for intricacies like hills, closed roads, or traffic. Therefore, you may have to ultimately run the course at least once to determine if it is an acceptable route to use in the future.

In conclusion

Route design is and should be an important aspect of your run planning. Poorly planned routes can cause problems with safety and may result in your having to wait for traffic or other interruptions, depending on the environment in which you run. As a runner, you should be cognizant of several factors when planning your run such as traffic, weather, or running surface, and design a route that minimizes interruptions and allows you the most favorable running conditions. Depending on your running goals, you may have several different routes to utilize, and having multiple options can ensure that no matter the situation, you have a route available that allows you to get your run accomplished.

Chapter 6: Understand the weather

One nice thing about running is that it can be done indoors or outdoors. As such, during those times that weather can be extreme you can simply choose to run indoors if adequate equipment or facilities are available. However, many runners claim that indoor workouts quickly become boring as there is little scenery change. Because you have the option of running outdoors, understanding the intricacies of the weather can help you have a more productive run. Weather can influence your runs in many ways, from the clothing you wear to the degree of exertion you feel. And, in the cases of extreme weather such as rain or a hot summer sun, failure to plan adequately for the weather can adversely affect your total run time. It is also important to understand that weather can actually be dangerous for you as a runner, such as if you expose too much skin during cold, windy runs or if you run during the middle of the day on a hot, humid afternoon. Therefore, this chapter will focus on outlining the various aspects of weather that can have an influence on your runs, such as radiation, heat index, wind chill, and dew point. A better understanding of weather can help ensure that your runs are productive while also ensuring that you are properly prepared against the sometimes-harsh effects of weather.

Types of weather

From a practical aspect, weather's primary influence on running centers around a safety aspect. If you run in hot weather and aren't able to cool yourself properly by either wearing minimal clothing or ensuring adequate hydration, you increase the risk of heat-related illnesses such as heat exhaustion. Similarly, if you run in extremely cold and/or windy conditions you might have a risk of frostbite, or potentially an injury resulting from slipping on ice. Severe injuries or illness such as heat stroke or a moderate to severe ankle sprain can result in no running activity for weeks or months, so it is essential that you work to minimize your risk of running in certain weather conditions.

Though injuries are a primary concern, your running ability can also be affected by weather. Running in hot, humid weather can significantly diminish your energy as well as your body's fluid levels, thereby requiring a careful monitoring of fluid intake to prevent dehydration. Running in rain can saturate clothing and make that clothing both heavier as well as somewhat uncomfortable. As a result, a simple shift in your schedule or attire can often allow you to have a more enjoyable run. This might occur by avoiding the mid-day sun and high temperatures, or wearing clothing that has minimal capability to absorb sweat.

Solar Radiation

You may have heard a sort of runner's mantra that cool weather is fantastic and warm weather is not bad. What you likely won't hear is that hot weather is either fantastic or even 'not bad'. Hot weather can be miserable for your runs, and attempting to avoid hot weather can often be a factor in when and where you run.

First, understand a little about the sun's position. Assuming that you are running on a clear day, the curvature of the earth means that the sun's radiation affects you differently throughout the day. From late morning to late afternoon, or approximately 10a.m. to 3-4p.m. the sun's rays will be most direct, depending somewhat upon what months you run. The most intense time point during this range is around noon as the sun approaches a 90 degree angle from the surface of the earth. Consequently, the intensity of solar radiation that your body absorbs is highest during this time, meaning that your body will be absorbing the maximal amount of radiation as well, in turn further elevating your body's temperature. This can result in greater skin temperature as well as a reduction in maximal effort, as has been shown scientifically (Otani Kaya Tamaki Effect of solar radiation on endurance EJAP 2016). What this research shows is that exercising during periods of peak solar radiation (i.e. most direct sunlight) can negatively affect your workload, translating quite simply as you not being able to run as far as if the sun was less of a factor. These results indicate that direct sunlight can have a significant influence on your run. When you combine the heat produced by your body while running along with the solar radiation that you absorb during mid-morning to mid-afternoon, it can set you up for not only a miserable run but also a potentially dangerous run if you are not taking adequate measure to protect yourself from the heat.

Not only is elevated body temperature a risk, but because the sun's radiation is most direct during this time, sunburn risk is also most likely increased.

Therefore, it is important that you take measures to protect yourself as well as your skin during this time. There is somewhat of a catch-22 situation here, as reducing sunburn risk means that you will need to cover your skin, while heat-illness risk can be reduced if you *expose* your skin and allow body heat to be removed by the air. If you must run during those times of the day that the sun's radiation is most intense, ensure that you have adequate skin exposure and protect your skin with a proper sunblock.

Based on the effects of the sun, to maximize your run productivity you may wish to run in the mornings or evenings when the sun's rays are less direct, at least during the hot times of the year. If you run when the sun's radiation is strong, you will likely fatigue early and feel out-of-shape or as though you are regressing in your fitness level, which is not necessarily true. Rather, your body may be having to work much harder due to the presence of strong solar radiation that can work to increase your body temperature above and beyond that generated from your body's activity level.

Dew point

You're probably looking at the words 'dew point' and wondering either what the heck it is or what it's doing in a running book. To assuage your concern, let me first ask you – are you familiar with humidity? Most likely you are, and you are probably familiar with how miserable the humidity can make you feel during a run. Because you are familiar with humidity, you may not realize it but you are already referencing the dew point when you talk about humidity. In fact, you might be surprised to learn that humidity is actually *determined* in large part by the dew point itself. To help you understand what the dew point is as well as the way in which it can affect 'how it feels' outside, we need to look a bit deeper into how moisture in the air can affect us.

You already know that air holds moisture in the form of water vapor. You may also know that air can only hold so much moisture, up to a point at which it becomes *saturated* with moisture. When saturation occurs, the air can hold no more water and the moisture begins to condense, or form condensation, on surfaces such as windows or potentially in the form of rainfall.

The temperature of the air determines how much moisture it can hold. Cold air can hold less moisture than warm air. This is why you may have heard that cold air is 'dryer' than warm air. The reason the air feels dryer is because there is inherently less water in the air than in the same amount of warm air. For example, if you opened a one-quart jar in the winter and let cold air in, and then did it again in the summer, the volume of air in the jar is the same. However, the total amount of moisture in the winter jar will be less because – as stated – cold air holds less moisture. So the amount of water in warm air is higher than the amount of moisture in the same amount of cold air, simply because warm air can hold more moisture.

Why does this matter? Well, let's look at what dew point is in order to explain that. Dew point is the temperature (typically read in Fahrenheit in the United States) at which the air itself will be saturated with water vapor. When the temperature falls to a level that matches the dew point, the water vapor present in the air begins to condense on any surface it can find. At this point – when the dew point and temperature are equal – the air is saturated and the *relative humidity* is said to be 100%. In other words, the air is holding 100% of the moisture it can hold at that particular temperature. Consequently, colder air will be associated with lower dew points while warmer air will have higher dew points as a result of being able to hold more water.

An example would probably be relevant here. If the dew point is 72 degrees Fahrenheit (72F) and the air temperature is 77F during the early morning, the air is not saturated because the two markers are not

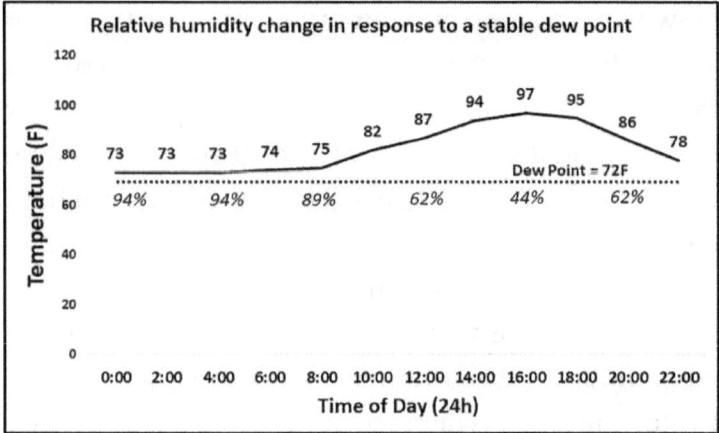

Relative humidity change in response to a stable dew point

As shown in this example, an increase in temperature during the afternoon hours results in falling humidity values (shown below the dashed line) despite no change in the dew point as the day progresses.

equal. Therefore, the relative humidity is not 100% as it can still hold more water. But unlike temperature, dew points do not usually change much during the day. Therefore, as the temperature begins to increase throughout the morning, the humidity actually *decreases* since the temperature is getting further away from the dew point. Remember, warmer air can hold more moisture than cooler air, so as the air temperature rises, the air's ability to hold moisture also increases. Using our example, with a dew point of 72F, as the temperature rises from 77F to 80F to 85F, the increasingly warmer air can hold more moisture despite no change in dew point. What you will see is a subsequent decrease in the reported humidity value as a result.

Calculating the actual humidity is a bit technical, as it involves vapor pressure and saturation pressure which are beyond the scope of this book. You can, however, find humidity (and dew point) calculators online that can perform this operation for you.

A lay person's way of thinking of humidity might be to say "If the dew point is 72F and the temperature is 80F, approximately what percent of the way is the temperature towards reaching full saturation of the air?" Well, using the earlier scenario, if the dew point is 72F and the air temperature was also 72F, you would know that the relative humidity would be 100%. Since the air temperature is actually higher (80F) in this new example, that percent relative humidity starts falling away from 100%, and at 80F lands around 74% humidity. In other words, the air temperature is 74% of the way to being saturated, and to get to 100% the air temperature needs to fall 8F more to increase the humidity by 26%. If the temperature keeps increasing, the humidity will continue to fall since the temperature moves further and further away from allowing for 100% saturation, or 72F (i.e. the dew point).

So why does this all matter for you as a runner? The problem with dew point for anyone performing activity outside in what are considered humid climates (e.g. gulf coast, southeast US, etc.) is that in the summer when the air is warm and can hold more moisture, the dew points will get much higher than what you will find in the winter or colder months. Other states with lower dew points in the summer – such as those in the Western US – still get high temperatures, but the air is much dryer and so the air feels less 'humid'.

High dew points can be problematic as the increased moisture in the air can affect how well sweat evaporates from your skin. If the air is nearly saturated, (i.e. when the temperature is near the dew point) it is not going to be very quick to evaporate the additional moisture from your skin. Consequently, sweat will drip down your skin rather than quickly evaporating, which in turn will reduce your body's cooling process. Conversely, in dry climates with much lower dew points the sweat has much more potential to evaporate due to the lower relative humidity of the air, particularly during the hotter times of the day.

Looking back to our earlier discussion of solar radiation, we outlined how avoiding runs during the heat of the mid-day summer afternoon can benefit you as a runner. That kind of thinking is somewhat correct, as you will avoid the effects of solar radiation. However, if you run during the early mornings you will have the situation of lower temperatures that are often hovering around the dew point. And if you will be running in a climate with high (e.g. < 70F) dew points, it can be problematic for your runs as the high relative humidity can make for a very 'muggy' run. Yet, as the temperature rises and you see a subsequent decrease in the humidity, the solar radiation will increase the rate at which body heat develops. Therefore, you may have to work to find a 'happy medium' between a humid run and a very hot run during certain months of the year.

Understand that dew point – much like solar radiation – are really only an issue for runners in the summer, as cold weather renders the dew point relatively meaningless. If, for example, you went for a run when it was sunny with an air temperature of 52F and a dew point of 50F, the humidity would be 93%. We all know that running in 52 degree weather is excellent running weather, and the humidity would actually have no real impact on our running capacity. On the other hand, if the air temperature was 93 and the dew point was 74 (humidity 53%), despite the relatively low humidity level you'd quickly realize that the run would be much less favorable compared to the colder run, despite its higher humidity level.

Unlike other measures of comfort such as heat index (discussed later), there is no accepted indicator of dew point specific to adjusting outside activity levels. Some have developed independent dew point

Dew Point	Perception
76+	Oppressive
71-75	Miserable
66-70	Uncomfortable
61-65	Annoying
56-60	Acceptable
<55	Outstanding

An example of a dew point scale based on the perception of how it feels to be outside

'comfort zones', but these are somewhat arbitrary and vary widely. Most often, these zones will show that any dew point above 70F is 'extremely uncomfortable' or similar, and anything above the mid-70's requires a cessation of activity. What this means is that going for a run when the dew point is over 70F is interpreted as being 'extremely uncomfortable'. However, many people live in areas where a 70F dew point is a daily occurrence during the summer months, rendering such an interpretation of high dew points to be quite subjective in nature. Similarly, an individual coming from a desert climate to run in one of the southeast states may find a 66F dew point unbearably hot in June, while that same dew point may make the air feel almost cool to a local individual who is used to dew points in the mid-70s. While these hypothetical comfort zones have merit, they are somewhat dependent upon each individual's personal tolerance. I will add that I once read that if the sum of the dew point and temperature is less than 100, it is outstanding running weather. However, even this arbitrary scale is somewhat dependent upon the climate that the runner is used to, and therefore cannot be expected to hold true for all runners.

Relative humidity

As you can now understand, that old adage of "it's not the heat, it's the humidity" isn't quite correct. Rather, it should read "It's not the heat, it's not the humidity, *it's the dew point*". Regardless, now that you have been exposed to dew point we can look briefly at relative humidity. I say briefly because as you now know, relative humidity is really nothing more than an indicator of how close the air temperature is to the dew point. Nevertheless, 'humidity' is often represented incorrectly as an indicator of the level of moisture in the air.

In actuality, we have to be careful to say *relative* humidity, since simply saying 'humidity' is indicative of absolute humidity – the total amount of water vapor present in a given volume. However, absolute humidity does not factor in temperature. Therefore relative humidity is the term used to represent the ratio between air temperature and dew point. As shown earlier, high humidity can be very mild such as when occurring in association with cold temperatures, or miserable when occurring in conjunction with high temperatures. As the ratio of temperature and dew point begin to separate, the relative humidity decreases, while as the values of temperature and dew point approach each other, relative humidity increases.

What you have likely recognized is that as the relative humidity rises, the comfort of running decreases proportionally. This is due to the fact that as the air approaches saturation there is less of a likelihood for the sweat on your skin to be evaporated, and evaporation of sweat is the process by which your body most effectively cools itself. In the absence of wind, evaporation occurs rather slowly in higher-humidity conditions. But, as air speed increases, the amount of air coming across the skin increases as well, thereby allowing more moisture to be removed from the skin. Therefore, running on a windy day will result in better body cooling as the air is able to remove more sweat (and thereby 'heat') from your body. Conversely, sitting down on a hot, calm day immediately after your run ends would result in minimal body cooling due to the fact that very little air is reaching your skin to help evaporate the sweat. On such days, try to continue to walk or stand in front of a fan to help maximize the amount of air that moves across your skin.

As humid air exhibits a diminished ability to hold water – and therefore evaporate sweat – a runner should be aware that he or she will likely be sweating to a very high degree. Consequently, the runner's clothing will absorb much of the sweat, in turn increasing both the overall weight of the clothing (due to the absorbed sweat) as well as increasing the possibility for chafing due to the potential friction generated in areas like the armpit or groin as a result of the saturated clothing. Therefore, reflecting back to the earlier chapter on equipment, clothing that is effective at 'wicking' sweat and minimizing the amount of sweat retained in clothing is certainly preferable, particularly when running on days with a high dew point.

Heat Index

One of the major summertime concerns when working or running outdoors in the heat is the *heat index*. The heat index is a value that is determined by both the air temperature and the relative humidity that indicates what the temperature feels like to the human body when the humidity is factored in. As discussed earlier, when the relative humidity rises, sweat cannot be evaporated as effectively from the skin. You still sweat the same, but during periods of higher relative humidity, sweat cannot be evaporated as efficiently from the body. Therefore, the body does not cool at the same rate as when there is low relative humidity, meaning that a high heat index – which results from high temperature and high humidity – feels much hotter to the body than the temperature itself may seem.

Rising humidity itself is not a problem necessarily. As we have shown, cold air and high relative humidity will likely have little influence on your runs. However when a high relative humidity is combined with a high temperature, the human body can suffer. As the sweat fails to evaporate adequately due to the high relative humidity, the body's temperature can increase, thereby setting up the opportunity for a severe heat-related illness such as heat stroke or heat exhaustion.

As the heat index value rises, recommendations to limit outdoor activity are often enacted. In such cases, running should be avoided during those periods of the day when high heat indexes occur – such as mid-to late-mornings or early afternoons during the summer. General recommendations suggest that as the heat index approaches 90F or above, outdoor activity should be limited in proportion to the rising heat index. And whereas heat index values are calculated using temperature readings taken in the shade, being in direct sunlight can be even more problematic given the potential for solar radiation from the sun further increasing the temperature of anyone working or running in direct sunlight.

Be aware that although the air temperature itself may not seem excessively high, when combined with a high relative humidity a dangerous condition can arise. For example, look at the heat index chart listed below. When looking at the humidity (top row) and comparing it to the air temperature (left column), you will see that even a temperature of 84F, when combined with a relative humidity value of 80%, puts the heat index at 94F. This heat index value is ten

	% Relative Humidity												
	40	45	50	55	60	65	70	75	80	85	90	95	100
110	136												
108	130	137											
106	124	130	137										
104	119	124	131	137									
102	114	119	124	130	137								
100	109	114	118	124	129	136							
98	105	109	113	117	123	128	134						
96	101	104	108	112	116	121	126	132					
94	97	100	103	106	110	114	119	124	129	135			
92	94	96	99	101	105	108	112	116	121	126	131		
90	91	93	95	97	100	103	106	109	113	117	122	127	132
88	88	89	91	93	95	98	100	103	106	110	113	117	121
86	85	87	88	89	91	93	95	97	100	102	105	108	112
84	83	84	85	86	88	89	90	92	94	96	98	100	103
82	81	82	83	84	84	85	86	88	89	90	91	93	95
80	80	80	81	81	82	82	83	84	84	85	86	86	87

(Air Temperature (F) — left axis label)

Heat index values relative to temperature and humidity. Darker shading represents increasing danger to individuals who are outside when the heat index is at those particular values.

degrees higher than the relatively tolerable air temperature of 84F. Consequently, at a seemingly mild air temperature of 84F an outdoor runner must take caution to prevent against heat illnesses.

Wind Chill

Similar to the heat index, the wind chill is a value calculated from two separate weather factors: air temperature and wind speed. Wind chill is a value that represents how heat is removed from the body faster due to the passing of cold air across the skin. Much like how solar radiation can increase the rate at which the body heats up, wind can be effective at increasing the cooling rate of the body as it helps remove body heat as the wind passes over the skin. In many conditions, wind is beneficial for cooling; however, when wind is combined with low air temperatures, the amount of cooling that occurs can become dangerous.

When the air temperature drops below 40F, runners should be wary of the wind chill. This means that exposed skin should be covered in order to prevent unnecessary heat loss, as in cold weather as much heat as possible should be retained. To outline the effect of wind chill, look at the chart below. As evident on the chart, when the wind is calm there is no change in wind chill since the lack of moving air does not remove heat faster from the body. However, as the wind speed (top row) increases, the wind chill value decreases proportionally. For example, a 15 mile per hour wind at 40F cools the body as if it were 32F outside. This can be particularly dangerous for runners if exposed skin is left uncovered, as tissue damage can occur. Furthermore, when running into a headwind, you should add your running speed to the existing wind speed, as your motion generates

Wind Speed (mph)												
Air Temperature (F)	5	10	15	20	25	30	35	40	45	50	55	60
40	36	34	32	30	29	28	28	27	26	26	25	25
35	31	27	25	24	23	22	21	20	19	19	18	17
30	25	21	19	17	16	15	14	13	12	12	11	10
25	19	15	13	11	9	8	7	6	5	4	4	3
20	13	9	6	4	3	1	0	-1	-2	-3	-3	-4
15	7	3	0	-2	-4	-5	-7	-8	-9	-10	-11	-11
10	1	-4	-7	-9	-11	-12	-14	-15	-16	-17	-18	-19
5	-5	-10	-13	-15	-17	-19	-21	-22	-23	-24	-25	-26
0	-11	-16	-19	-22	-24	-26	-27	-29	-30	-31	-32	-33
-5	-16	-22	-26	-29	-31	-33	-34	-36	-37	-38	-39	-40
-10	-22	-28	-32	-35	-37	-39	-41	-43	-44	-45	-46	-48
-15	-28	-35	-39	-42	-44	-46	-48	-50	-51	-52	-54	-55
-20	-34	-41	-45	-48	-51	-53	-55	-57	-58	-60	-61	-62
-25	-40	-47	-51	-55	-58	-60	-62	-64	-65	-67	-68	-69
-30	-46	-53	-58	-61	-64	-67	-69	-71	-72	-74	-75	-76
-35	-52	-59	-65	-68	-71	-73	-76	-78	-79	-81	-82	-84

Wind chill values based on wind speed and temperature. Darker shading represents an increasing risk of frostbite for exposed skin at those particular values.

even higher airflow speeds across your skin. For example, if you are running at 7mph into a 10mph headwind, the air is moving across your skin at 17mph, thereby resulting in an even lower wind chill than shown on a chart. As such, when running in cold weather it is imperative that you cover skin that is exposed unnecessarily so as to prevent that skin from losing unnecessary heat.

Lightning

Injuries from heat and cold are largely avoidable, even when detected during the early stages of the condition. Lightning, however, may give no warning and can result in death. Though one might think that it can be left unsaid, lightning is an extremely dangerous situation for runners, and reducing the possibility of a lightning strike typically means either getting a run in well before a storm is in the vicinity, or running indoor during times of heightened risk. While it might seem somewhat ridiculous to mention that lightning is an issue for runners given that there is typically a warning in the way of evidence of a developing storm, lightning can strike as far as 10 miles out from a storm. This is particularly important for runners, who often run outdoors on long stretches of flat road which in turn can make them susceptible to a lightning strike. Furthermore, as runners often run alone, there is little to no chance for immediate help in the event of a lightning strike, leaving the runner no real option for life-saving first aid.

Because of the danger associated with lightning, you should always check the weather forecast as well as radar prior to starting your run. Several real-time phone radar apps are available that will show you the intensity, direction, and sometimes even predicted arrival times of storms, and you should be wary of starting outdoor running activity that could put you in the vicinity of any storm. If there is a chance for a storm to develop, you should either outline a running course that makes several passes near a safe shelter (e.g. home, indoor facility, etc.), wait until the storm has passed, or until the threat of a storm diminishes.

In conclusion

Although weather can vary widely both prior to and during your runs, there are several conditions that can make a day's run dangerous or even life-threatening. During those times of the year that the temperature can become unbearably hot, runners should consider early-morning runs or at minimum ensure that they are making sound decisions regarding clothing, sunscreen, and skin exposure. Even in less-than-ideal weather, proper preparation can help ensure that weather does not negatively influence your running activity. Preparation requires monitoring weather reports and dressing appropriately for the weather which you will be encountering as a runner. For those times of the year when weather can be oppressive, such as might occur during the hot summer months, you may have to take extra precautions to ensure your safety from the weather. And, you will have to plan carefully to ensure that you can still have an enjoyable run despite the weather conditions.

Chapter 7: Take care of your injuries

Not much can stop progress in your running plan quite like an injury. Whether it be a mild sprain or an overuse injury, suffering from a running-related injury requires proper care in order to get you back to your pre-injury running ability. Given what the body goes through in response to running activity, you should *expect* an injury of some kind eventually. Hopefully you will experience nothing more than a minor muscle strain or even a friction injury like a blister. Regardless of the cause, your focus should be on making sure that the injury heals properly in order to ensure that the injury itself has fully healed and also prevent a future recurrence.

When it comes to running, the majority of injuries that you will experience can be lumped into either friction-based injury – such as blisters or chafing – or orthopedic injuries that affect bones, muscles, and/or joints. Regardless of the cause, injuries cause cellular damage that in turn releases chemicals called *mediators* that are designed to alert the body to the presence of an injury and in turn trigger healing. During the healing process the body works to repair the damaged tissue and effectively return it to pre-injury status. This requires a series of processes that remove damaged tissue and generates new tissue over time. Continued physical stresses to the tissue while under repair during this time period can delay the healing process. Therefore, it is important for runners to be able to recognize the difference between an injury that generates "soreness" versus an injury that needs to be given time to properly heal.

For example, if you conduct a hill workout for the first time in six months, you will certainly feel the consequences in your legs for the next few days, specifically in the way of soreness. This should not be considered a true 'injury' and is actually the normal response to a strenuous workout. However, if while doing those hill workouts you felt a sudden, sharp pain in your calf, there's a pretty good chance that you suffered an injury to a muscle or tendon. Consequently, you will need to let the tissue heal properly in order to return to your normal running plan. While injuries can certainly interfere with your running, the care and treatment of injuries is not the focus of this book, and I recommend that you look into one of the several available books on the topic of running injuries.

Your body will tell you when something is wrong. In fact, that's really the purpose of pain, numbness, tingling, etc. – to inform you that something is wrong with an area of your body and needs your attention. Yes, pain hurts, and yes, pain can get in the way of your training, but it is critical that you take the time to deal with the source of the pain so that the tissue can heal and you can return to your normal running routine.

Not all injuries require a complete cessation of running activity. In fact, many injury care professionals will have you back on a modified running plan well before the injury is fully healed. Doing so helps ensure that you limit what is called *deconditioning.* Deconditioning occurs when the gains that you have made as a result of your running – such as an increase in speed or VO2max – diminish due to a removal of the stresses (i.e. running) that invoked the original gains. For example, if you run consistently for six months and your aerobic fitness measurement increases from 38 to 47, you could easily claim that your fitness has increased. However, if you are then injured in a car wreck and you are unable to run for six weeks, upon finally recovering enough to go for a run you may find that your VO2max has dropped back down to 40. This in effect represents what happens in response to deconditioning. The challenge is to find other activities to perform which can limit the degree of deconditioning that you might experience. However, the type of activity you can continue to perform is largely dependent upon the type and location of injury you have suffered, and it is always recommended that you receive professional care for any injury you incur, especially prior to returning to your running activity.

Friction injuries

One of the most likely injuries that you will suffer will be some sort of friction wound. These type of wounds can include blisters, chafing, callous formation, or even an occasional raw nipple or two. In most cases, friction wounds are relatively minor on the injury scale and require only a bit of protection through the use of a dressing, after which you typically can continue on with your running plan. The thing to be aware of, however, is that you should look into the actual mechanism that caused the friction wound. For example, blisters on the feet are often caused by new or improperly-fit shoes. If a blister occurs in response to a new shoe, the 'break-in' phase of the shoe – that portion of time that you wear the shoe for a short time to allow it to form to your foot over time – will eventually allow the shoe to adapt to the intricacies of your particular foot. This is the very reason why you should never wear brand new shoes on the day of a race. Rather, wear them around the house for a few days and on a short run or two in order to allow them to adjust to your feet.

If a blister forms as a result of improperly-fit shoes, the obvious fix is to determine where the issue lies with the shoe. Is it too long? Too wide? Too small? In some cases, a slightly oversized shoe can be compensated for by wearing an additional pair of socks; however, the first line of defense is to ensure that you have a properly fitting shoe to begin with. The practice of improving the fit of a slightly large shoe by adding an additional sock is not recommended, as it can reduce the amount of air flow to your foot and thereby increase the amount of moisture retained in your socks and shoe. On the other hand, if the shoe feels too tight it can compress your foot and potentially cause a blister as well. As such, it is highly recommended that you find a properly fitting running shoe. Never expect that a tight shoe will "expand" adequately with continued use.

Chafing results from clothing rubbing repeatedly against the skin. Most often, the clothing has become damp with sweat which increases the amount of friction generated. The fact that certain fabrics such as cotton absorb and hold on to moisture is why running clothes should be light, thin and made from a type of material that "wicks" the sweat off of the skin and allows it to be evaporated faster. Shirts, shorts, and even socks now come in materials designed to remove moisture quickly and reduce the risk of chafing due to moisture. The groin area, nipples, underarms, and the feet are all areas subject to chafing, and it is important for a runner to find equipment that can help reduce the incidence of chafing. Depending on the time of year, a runner could become sweaty just minutes into a run, and an early onset of chafing can have drastic consequences during longer runs, eventually breaking the skin and causing bleeding in the area. And the more severe the chafing becomes, the longer the time frame for the injury to heal. Skin lubricants can help as well, but the first priority should be on finding effective run clothing to help prevent the initial incidence of chafing.

Besides pain, chafing injuries have a high potential for developing what is called a "broken" skin wound. Broken skin occurs when the skin itself is no longer intact and removes the protective barrier formed by healthy skin. This in turn allows pathogens such as bacteria to infiltrate an area, in turn heightening the risk of infection. Blisters are particularly unique when it comes to broken skin, as they can exist at a stage of either unbroken or broken skin, depending on the state of the blister. If, for example, a blister forms on your heel and 'pops' during your run, it can develop into a broken skin wound if enough skin layers are affected. This would in turn cause bleeding as well as a greater risk of infection. On the other hand, a blister that results in a simple formation of fluid underneath an outer layer will likely remain intact, thereby failing to 'break' the skin and minimizing the opportunity for infection.

Orthopedic injuries

While friction wounds are relatively minor, orthopedic (i.e. bone and muscle) injuries require much more attention. In running, most orthopedic-related injuries are going to occur below the waist as that is where the majority of force is placed upon the body. Foot stress fractures, ankle sprains, calf and hamstring strains, or hip pain are all relatively common in running and as mentioned earlier, at some point every runner should be expected to incur at least one of these injuries.

One of the fascinating things about the human body is that the harder you work it, the stronger it becomes. No material object you own has this kind of characteristic. Imagine your car becoming more efficient the harder you drive it, or your lawnmower blade becoming sharper every time it is used. Obviously, those two things can't happen. Yet, the more our bodies are subjected to strenuous activity the better it can perform. This is one of the inherent qualities of living tissue – the ability to adapt and change to the stresses imposed upon it.

Activities such as running expose the body to repetitive stress, which – when it occurs within reason – the body can easily handle. Sometimes, however, that level of stress either increases or becomes highly focused in one particular area. When this occurs, tissue gets damaged and we experience the resulting injury. If the injury occurs in muscle or tendon tissue, we experience a strain. Excessive force in a bone can trigger a fracture, while repetitive force over time can generate a stress fracture. Joint stresses can cause arthritis, meniscal damage, or a sprain. Regardless of the type of tissue affected, it is essential that you seek the assistance of a medical professional in order to properly diagnose and care for your injury.

As a runner, the important issue is to make sure that your injury is both recognized (by you) and diagnosed (by a medical professional). This ensures that a proper treatment plan is designed that will get you on the path to a full recovery. Some running-related injuries will allow you to continue without pause. Others can require a full cessation of running activity, even though the injury itself may not seem particularly debilitating. Unfortunately, many runners will decide to 'push through' an injury that they feel is not particularly painful, only to end up converting that same injury from relatively minor to somewhat severe in nature. Therefore, be sure to consult with a medical professional on any orthopedic injury. Avoid the temptation or suggestion to self-diagnose your injury on the internet, as something like a seemingly small knee injury could be anything from a tendon strain to a fracture to a meniscus injury.

In conclusion

Activities such as running expose the body to repetitive stress, which – when it occurs within reason – the body is capable of handling. Every once in a while, however, that level of stress either increases or becomes highly focused in one particular area, and tissue gets damaged. We see this as an injury.

Don't take any injury for granted as a runner. Friction injuries, though something that you may feel is just an issue of mind over matter, can make for miserable subsequent runs if not properly cared for. Always take time to treat any friction wound properly, and be sure to minimize the risk of potential infection. Similarly, orthopedic injuries must be evaluated quickly in order to prevent the possibility of further damage. If you take a few steps on a mildly sprained ankle, it may not really bother you at all. However, if you instead take 5,000 steps on that same sprained ankle during the course of a run, you can cause significant further injury and therefore delay the healing process for what would have originally been a relatively insignificant injury. When it comes to running-related injuries, I recommend that you always seek the care and/or advice of a medical professional, preferably one that has experience with running-related conditions.

Conclusion

Running can offer you a variety of positive benefits – better health, improved fitness, the exhilaration of being outdoors, and perhaps even a longer life. With that comes the effort and energy required to start, engage in, and finish your runs. When heading out the door for a run, you may have low motivation or even a bit of hesitation to put forth the energy needed for the run. This book was written with the intent to make you aware of potential ways to both enjoy running more and also get more out of your runs.

As I mentioned in the introduction, the premise of this book arose from various conversations with both new and experienced runners. I finally decided that I would interject my own experiences and training into the specific topics in order to provide a book that can help runners overcome some of the most common factors that negatively influence their running: lack of motivation, weather, equipment, and a few others. I hope that after having read this book you feel that you have a better understanding of these potential issues. Furthermore, I hope that you can use what you have learned in this book in order to stave off the negative consequences of many of the issues we discussed so as to ensure that you have an enjoyable run.

Running is a lifestyle, and no one will argue that running does not make you a healthier individual. Because of the obvious benefits that running brings with it, it is important that you continue to run and be physically active in general for as long as you can in life. Eliminating negative factors that can inhibit both your love of running as well as your ability to run are key in ensuring that you continue to enjoy running. I tried to outline for you in this book what I felt were many of the factors that can inhibit your ability to have an enjoyable run. By eliminating the negative, you will in turn accentuate the positive. This should be expected to result in a more fit, healthier you.

I wish you the best of luck in your future running adventures, and I look forward to the opportunity to see you out on the running paths.

Other published books written by Mark Knoblauch

In addition to *Seven Ways*, Mark has released five prior books, and is also working on several additional works. And, if you are interested in academic writing, be sure to watch for the release of his upcoming book detailing how to improve your professional writing skills.

Overcoming Ménière's. How changing your lifestyle can change your life.

ISBN# 978-1-7320674-7-9

Overcoming Ménière's provides the reader a detailed overview of Ménière's including the involved anatomy as well as the most recent research. By detailing his own Ménière's journey as well as what has worked for his own battle with Ménière's, Mark intends to provide other Ménière's sufferers a pathway which they themselves can following in order to find similar relief from the devastating effects of Ménière's disease.

Understanding BPPV. Outlining the causes and effects of Benign Paroxysmal Positional Vertigo

ISBN# 978-1-7320674-1-7

Benign Paroxysmal Positional Vertigo is a condition that triggers vertigo when the head is placed in a particular position. Furthermore, the vertigo ceases once the head is repositioned. Despite the somewhat forceful symptoms inherent to BPPV, the underlying cause of BPPV is relatively minor and can typically be fixed with a simple visit to a medical professional's office.

Because of his own experience with BPPV, Mark wrote *Understanding BPPV* so that everyone affected by this condition can have a solid resource guide outlining just what BPPV is, how it occurs, and how it is treated. Particular attention is focused on the anatomy of the ear, and how this anatomy is involved in generating the symptoms associated with BPPV. Mark also details the latest research into BPPV and provides an overview of the various diagnostic tests and treatments used to help BPPV patients in many cases get back to a vertigo-free life.

Essentials of Writing and Publishing your Self-Help Book

ISBN# 978-1-7320674-9-3

Some people elect to transform their own experiences and successes into a self-help book that outlines how they persevered through their difficult times. As a potential self-help book author yourself, you might be struggling to get started, get finished, or just need tips on how to finally get your advice and ideas onto bookstore shelves. *Essentials of Writing and Publishing Your Self-Help Book* is filled with information that will help walk you through the process of producing a quality self-help book. You'll be exposed to strategies that will help get you through the various stages of book production, gain insight into the options you have available for publication of your book, and review the individual steps and requirements necessary to get your advice from paper to a finished book.

Hidden down deep inside of us, we all have a book waiting to be written. The tips and techniques outlined in this book are designed to help you bring your ideas, successes, and lessons to life in the form of your own self-help book.

Outlining Tinnitus. A comprehensive guide to help you break free of the ringing in your ears.

ISBN: 978-1-7320674-2-4

The underlying cause of tinnitus has been described by researchers as one of the most controversial issues in medical science. Despite decades of intense research, the cure for tinnitus remains elusive. Consequently, millions of tinnitus sufferers are left susceptible to the frustration and annoyance brought about by the ever-present ringing in their ears. Mark Knoblauch has himself lived with tinnitus for over 15 years and understands the daily battles that occur in those individuals afflicted with tinnitus.

Now, despite still living with tinnitus daily, the high-pitched sound in his ear has become nothing more than an afterthought thanks to a dedicated treatment plan. And the success he had in addressing his own tinnitus drove him to write Outlining Tinnitus. This book is designed to serve as an all-inclusive guide for those individuals who suffer from tinnitus as well as those who live with or know someone suffering. Topics such as the involved anatomy, suspected causes, available therapies and treatments, and effects on quality of life are all discussed along with many others in order to provide a comprehensive overview of what tinnitus is as well as how it can be effectively eliminated.

The art of efficiency. A guide for improving task management in the home to help maximize your leisure time

(ebook)

In a world that seemingly never has enough time, we are often unable to get everything done that we need to accomplish in a given time frame. Though we can take out our frustrations on the fact that there is just not enough time in our day, no matter what we want, we can't simply create more time. Therefore, we have to make the most of the time we do have and try to utilize our available time in the most efficient way possible.

When it comes to getting tasks done in the home, efficiency can be the key to determining how much free time we ultimately earn for ourselves. As we become more efficient, we can expect an improvement in the amount of time available for us to use as we please. This book highlights those tactics that I have found beneficial at helping me get my required tasks done at home in the most efficient way possible. More importantly, this book will show you how to structure your tasks based upon the required activity level (i.e. active vs. passive tasks), in turn being able to schedule your time-on-task in a way that results in significant time savings due to your improved efficiency at task completion.

Let others know!

If you found this or any of Mark's other books informative, *please take the time and post a review online*! Reviews help get exposure for the books and thereby improve the chances that others will be able to benefit from the material as well!

Image credits:

Shoe styles: Iakov Filimonov/shutterstock.com
Run clothing: Zilu8/shutterstock.com